FEARS, PHOBIAS & FANTASIES

FEARS, PHOBIAS & FANTASIES

UNDERSTANDING MENTAL HEALTH AND MENTAL ILLNESS

PROF. PATRICIA CASEY

CURRACH
BOOKS

First published in 2021 by

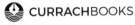
CURRACHBOOKS

Block 3b, Bracken Business Park, Bracken Road
Sandyford, Dublin 18.
www.currachbooks.com

ISBN: 978-1-78218-921-3

Set in Adobe Garamond Pro and Agenda
Cover and book design by Alba Esteban | Currach Books

Printed by L&C, Poland

To my husband John McGuiggan, for his unfailing
love, support, wisdom and great wit.

ACKNOWLEDGEMENTS

I am most grateful for the many people who willingly came forward and gave of their time to write the narratives, spread throughout this book. I am indebted to Garry O'Sullivan of Currach Books for placing his trust in my endeavour. Art Director Alba Esteban and copy-editor Fiona Biggs have been patient, professional, efficient and creative. Above all, they and Garry have been a pleasure to work with and their patience and creativity is greatly appreciated. My son James McGuiggan was invaluable in helping me to remove jargon and write in a style that faced the public rather than mental health professionals.

CONTENTS

Foreword

Mental health is complicated and mental health issues can affect all of us from time to time. For some people, their whole lives are changed. Traditionally the knowledge and power around mental health has been held by the physician and, more recently, by other mental health professionals. It is only over the last twenty years or so that the general public has become more informed about mental health issues. This book, by one of Ireland's foremost consultant psychiatrists, is a welcome addition to the canon of knowledge.

Notwithstanding her expertise as a consultant medical psychiatrist Professor Casey has not shied away from the more controversial issues of modern discourse. For centuries advocates have argued the nature/nurture debate to find valid cause for many of the conditions described in this book. Something of a truce appears to have been called with a tacit agreement that both nature and nurture can contribute to causation. Language is also a vexed question. Terms such as patient, client, service user, mental illness, mental ill health and disease, are espoused, adopted and abandoned by various factions in the intellectual war.

Issues such as the role of psychiatry in society have also been highlighted. Does psychiatry work for the greater good or for the benevolence of the individual? How is psychiatry used to control (and/or protect) society? Does psychiatry have the monopoly on mental ill health? How do other disciplines, such as psychology and sociology, fit into the equation?

Concurrent themes have also emerged concerning stigma and discrimination and the potential for recovery. Of particular importance is the emerging role of the individual and their family. Medicine in general and psychiatry in particular has shifted its stance from the doctor/patient relationship, based on an inequality of knowledge and power, to one based solidly on the sharing of knowledge and power reflected in a partnership approach. The 'doctor knows best' ethos is now (with exceptions in the case of involuntary admissions) no longer an acceptable working arrangement.

In fact, many of the underlying principles and practices of recovery-based mental health services are rooted in the concept that the individual can promote their own recovery by shaping their behaviour and taking control of their own life. Recovery comes from within and the role of modern mental health care is to provide a safe environment for recovery to flourish. Such interventions may of necessity be formal such as, for example, the provision of residential services and interventions to the person in their own community in a timely fashion by appropriately trained professionals.

More informal services, such as those provided by voluntary bodies, family and the wider community, are increasingly recognised as significant enablers of, for example, the restoration of self-esteem, building healthy social relationships and allowing people to be seen as valued members of the community. The important role of the family as support is increasingly recognised. While many may become patients, clients or service users of a mental health system and its professional staff, they are fundamentally and firstly people with lived experience who share all of the same rights and obligations of their fellow citizens.

In most western democracies this rights-based community model of service delivery founded on a shared participation in recovery is espoused in national policies such as, in Ireland, *Planning for the Future* (1984), *A Vision for Change* (2006) and, more recently, *Sharing the Vision* (2020). Happily, and not before time, countries such as Ireland have shifted their patterns of mental health care from a traditional asylum one based on custodial and paternalistic care (not always to the humane standards one would hope for) to a model that supports people to remain in their own home and to seek supports to aid recovery in their own community.

Professor Casey's book is a welcome aid to the general public to allow it to learn more about mental health and ill health and be able to understand the complex dynamics at play when someone's mental health is challenged or seriously affected. We have a duty, as citizens and supporters of the greater good, not only to understand but appreciate and perhaps, in our own way, to contribute to the well-being and recovery of those who in previous times could have been condemned to a life of isolation and incarceration.

John Saunders
CEO, Shine - Supporting People
Affected by Mental Ill Health

Introduction

The stigma of mental illness has diminished significantly in recent years. It is commonplace now for celebrities to discuss their mental health problems in the pages of popular magazines, on TV and in other media. The public has likewise become more willing to admit to vulnerabilities and to mental health needs. Self-help books abound and the shelves of bookshops display material about conditions from gaming addiction, to schizophrenia to narcissism. Despite this proliferation their quality cannot be vouched for and this benchmarking is challenging.

The purpose of *Fears, Phobias and Fantasies: Understanding mental health and mental illness* is to provide a single reference book for those needing information on mental illness. It will also be a resource for those interested in the subject matter – secondary school students, people working in areas allied to psychiatry, such as social workers, and, most of all, the general public. As Sir Francis Bacon said, *scientia potentia est* (knowledge is power).

The structure of the book is to provide descriptions of the major groups of psychiatric conditions. Controversies, not least how mental illness can be distinguished from normal distress, are highlighted. Legal and ethical concerns are also discussed, particularly the issue of confidentiality and how it is applied and misapplied in current practice. Since most readers will have no idea what happens at a psychiatric consultation this is described in the early part of the book, as is the history of psychiatry as a specialty. This background aims to provide a context to current practice. Additional reading material is suggested to amplify the chapters.

Useful resources are also listed, and these include details of YouTube content and other accessible materials, along with contact information for support organisations.

I am most indebted to all of those who wrote of their experience of living with a mental health condition. The contributions of those who have a loved one with a mental illness are both poignant and enriching. The response to my request for contributors, through Shine (a support organisation) was overwhelming and positive. Most opted to do this anonymously, while a few used initials, pseudonyms or their own name. These contributions give a reality to what could have been viewed as a theoretical detached account of mental illness. For most readers I believe the voice of these contributors will be the most helpful and illuminating part of the book Thank you all, from the bottom of my heart. I also wish to express my deep gratitude to Mr John Saunders, CEO of Shine, for his immediate and enthusiastic response to my request for contributors.

It is always difficult to convey complex mental health and illness information in a language that is comprehensible to those not trained in this area. In order to ensure that the writing can be understood, I have removed jargon, and where it has been used, I have attempted to explain the terms.

I was also mindful of the dangers inherent in writing a book such as this. Undoubtedly there will be some who will object to my use of the word 'patient' rather than 'service user' or 'client'. The rationale for this is explained on page 47. A more worrisome problem is that some may use this book to self-diagnose. This would be ill-advised. A book cannot replace a person-to-person consultation, although it can amplify the person's understanding of their own condition and also that of their family and close contacts. Some may also wonder why this book did not deal with child mental health, now a major problem in Ireland. Such a book is required, but as an adult psychiatrist I would have been outside my area of expertise, so I will leave that to one of my esteemed child psychiatrist colleagues to pursue.

This is the first book of its kind in Ireland. I trust that the material between the covers of this book will give hope and healing to those with mental health problems. It may also assist in enlightening attitudes to mental illness and in highlighting the need for continuing development of our mental health services.

1

History and Definition of Mental Illness

HISTORICAL PERSPECTIVES

In ancient times people thought of 'madness' as a punishment from the gods. The First Book of Samuel tells how King Saul was afflicted by madness after he neglected his duties to God. He slaughtered 85 priests at Nob in his state of illness, and David played the harp to soothe him.

Hippocrates (460–377 BC), a famous Greek physician, did not subscribe to the idea that mental illness was due to demonic possession or divine retribution, but rather took a physical view of it. He believed that it was due to imbalances in the four 'humours' of the body, namely black bile, yellow bile, phlegm and blood. The Roman physician Galen (129–200) developed this theory further. These ideas were also incorporated into Islamic medicine by the great physician and polymath Avicenna (980–1037).

Associations between humours, temperament and mental illness

Yellow bile, the first of the four humours, was associated with the gall bladder. It was believed that this contributed to the choleric or easily angered temperament.

Black bile was associated with the spleen, and this humour was believed to contribute to the melancholic or despondent temperament.

Blood was associated with the liver and was believed to contribute to the sanguine, courteous and optimistic temperament.

Phlegm was associated with the lungs and was believed to contribute to the phlegmatic or calm temperament.

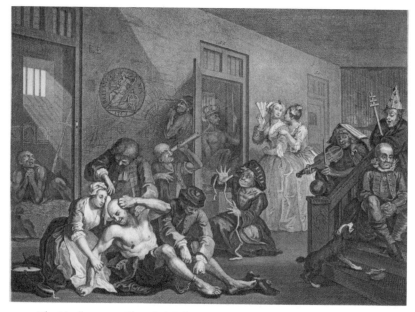

The Madhouse — Plate 8, *A Rake's Progress*, Engraving, William Hogarth.

In those early days, treatments such as purges, enemas and bloodletting were developed to release these humours from the ill person.

In the Middle Ages, 'madness' was again considered to be a moral disorder, the result of demonic possession or witchcraft. Sometimes it was managed by punishment, at others by exorcism. Some people, especially those believed to be witches, were hunted down and executed. Many of the mentally ill became vagrants, with some finding sanctuary at monasteries. In London, Bedlam was the first hospital for mentally ill paupers. It was built initially as a convent and later as a centre for the collection of alms for the Crusader church. The first definite record that it was housing the mentally ill was in 1403, but it may have been doing so since 1377. From 1720 to 1779 Bedlam allowed the rich to come and see the inmates, not so much for entertainment, but so as to generate compassion and therefrom, donations. It was believed that these spectacles might also offer cautionary advice against immoral living. A painting by Hogarth, *The Madhouse*, from the series titled *A Rake's Progress* (1732–34), captures the scene in Bedlam at this time.

Daniel Defoe (1660–1731), the author of *Robinson Crusoe*, was a leading campaigner for better facilities for those with mental illness, irrespective of their income, and he highlighted the atrocious conditions in the institutions for the insane, which by then were flourishing. These were mainly private, and there were few facilities for the poor with mental illness.

Jonathan Swift was one of the governors of the Bethlehem Hospital (also called Bethlem or Bedlam), in London. He governed the hospital from 1714 until his return to Dublin as Dean of St Patrick's Cathedral. His commitment to the mentally ill, harnessed by his role in the Bethlehem Hospital, ultimately resulted in his founding St Patrick's Psychiatric Hospital in Dublin in 1757. As a private institution, it was for the wealthy. However, two years later, St Brendan's Hospital was built in Grangegorman, on the north side of Dublin, and this expanded, for the first time, treatment and care to the poor. The plight of this group was starkly illustrated by the Right Honourable Denis Browne, an MP for Mayo, when he gave evidence to the Select Committee on the Lunatic Poor of Ireland, established by Robert Peel in 1817. He reported that 'When a strong young man or woman get the complaint, the only way they [the family] have to manage is by making a hole in the floor of the cabin not high enough for the person to stand up in, with a crib over it to prevent his getting up, the hole is about five feet deep, and they give the wretched being his food there, and there he generally dies' (Kelly, 2017).

Thereafter other asylums sprung up, and ultimately every county in Ireland had its psychiatric institution. They quickly exceeded their capacity, however, and while the initial intentions were good, the results, due to overcrowding and a lack of any therapeutic facilities, were dismal.

The word 'psychiatry' was first coined by Dr Johann Christian Reil in Germany in 1808. It is derived from two Greek words, *psukhe* (soul and mind) and *iatros* (healer), and so literally translates as 'healing of the soul/mind'. A psychiatrist, then, is one who heals the soul/mind. Until that time, mental illness, formally referred to as 'madness', 'lunacy' or 'insanity', was viewed as representing a moral or religious deficit. However, this point marked the start of a gradual change in perspective; instead of being viewed as a manifestation of evil, it began to be seen as an illness.

Not just Britain and Ireland, but Europe more generally witnessed the opening of hospitals to house the mentally ill towards the end of the 18th century. One of the largest was the Pitié-Salpêtrière Hospital in Paris, which housed over 10,000 inmates. These included the mentally ill but also vagrants, prostitutes and prisoners: the purpose of the Salpêtrière, as was the case for many asylums at this time, was not so much to cure the mentally ill as to protect public order by locking away disruptive undesirables. There, one day in 1792, the physician Philippe Pinel removed the manacles from more than 50 patients described as manic, and instituted a more humane approach to treatment called moral therapy. At the same time in York, England, a Quaker family, the Tukes, opened the York Retreat in 1796 and also used moral therapy. This consisted of treating the patients kindly, having them meet with non-ill people for conversations, allowing visitors, and allowing patients to work on the farm or gardens and to attend religious services. This was a milestone on the way to the modern treatment of those with mental illness. It also led to a change in the attitudes of the public and the medical profession. From York, this approach spread to the US: Pennsylvania opened the Friend's Retreat in Frankford in 1817, and in Connecticut, Eli Todd opened the Hartford Retreat in 1822.

At the same time, one of Britain's longest-reigning monarchs, George III (1738–1820), was experiencing periodic episodes of acute mental illness (believed to have been bipolar mania). This may have influenced the growing understanding and compassion towards those with mental illness.

Dr Benjamin Rush, the American physician who introduced the idea that mental illness was a disease of the mind, rather than a weakness in the person or something stemming from demonic possession or evil, is widely accepted as the father of psychiatry. His *Observations and Inquiries upon the Diseases of the Mind* (1812) was the first textbook of psychiatry. This work finally brought psychiatry within the ambit of medicine and gave psychiatrists the medical identity they enjoy to this day

PSYCHIATRY, PSYCHOLOGY AND OTHER DISCIPLINES

A profession with a distinct but related history to psychiatry is psychology. Psychiatrists and psychologists are often confused in the popular mind. Psychiatrists first become doctors and then train in the specialty of psychiatry. They deal with complex mental health problems and can prescribe medication or use talking and behavioural treatments. Their main therapeutic focus is severe mental illness such as schizophrenia, bipolar disorder and severe depressive illness. Their training takes place over approximately 10 years. Psychologists obtain a primary degree in psychology and then specialise in clinical psychology to PhD level under supervision. They cannot prescribe medication but instead use talking and behavioural therapies. Their training is approximately seven years. They most often treat anxiety, mild depressive disorders and behavioural conditions. Both professions work closely together in psychiatric multidisciplinary teams, often focusing on different aspects of the person's mental health condition.

The first involvement of psychologists in therapy occurred in the US in the early 1900s, when a number of child guidance clinics were established, and they employed psychologists to provide evaluation and treatment. However, their role as therapists increased significantly after the Second World War, as they moved into treating those affected by the war. By the 1960s the writings of some of these psychologists helped develop behavioural therapy and, subsequently, cognitive behavioural therapy (CBT). Since then psychologists have played a key role in these advances. One of the more recent examples is dialectical behaviour therapy ((DBT), developed by Marsha Linehan in the US in the late 1980s, now the treatment of choice for those who engage in repeated self-harm and have a diagnosis of emotionally unstable personality disorder (EUPD) (see Chapter 10), and this is supported by a significant number of published studies.

A further revolution, beginning in the 1980s, occurred when psychiatrists moved away from the traditional psychiatric hospitals (known as asylums and regarded with some prejudice) and began to work in psychiatric units located in general hospitals. In addition, the subspecialty known as liaison psychiatry began to develop. Liaison psychiatry refers to the management of mental health problems linked to physical illnesses. The first liaison psychiatrist in Ireland was Professor John Sheehan, appointed to the Mater Misericordiae University Hospital in Dublin in 1994. The presence of psychiatrists working shoulder to shoulder with cardiologists, transplant teams, oncologists and all the specialties has greatly enhanced the respect accorded to psychiatry, which until then had tended to be disparaged by other specialties. In a similar vein, psychologists now also work closely with physicians and surgeons as interventions become more complex and their psychological implications are increasingly appreciated.

DEVELOPMENTS IN THE LATE 20TH CENTURY

The image of mental hospitals dotted round the country is embedded in the memories of those who grew up before the 1980s. They were located on the edges of towns: large, forbidding, red- or grey-bricked buildings, surrounded by large tracts of land and topped with chimneys that seemed to touch the sky. Separated from the rest of the world by their high walls, nobody would dare go near them, lest the over-curious met the same fate as those inside. During their peak in Ireland, in the 1950s, some 20,000 people were housed in institutions for the mentally ill.

These have now almost all been sold, often to hoteliers, and have been replaced by dedicated, specialist wards in general hospitals. People no longer need long-term care to the extent they did in the past, thanks to the treatments that have been developed in recent decades, particularly for severe mental illness. For the few who do need permanent care, this is provided in domestic units, usually houses, staffed by nurses and doctors with the goal of providing rehabilitation and eventually restoration to more independent living.

MODERN TREATMENTS – DRUGS AND PSYCHOLOGICAL THERAPIES

These new treatments began to emerge in the 1960s. The first antidepressant, iproniazide, was discovered by chance in 1952. This drug was originally used in the treatment of tuberculosis, but it was observed that those taking this medication, who would have been expected to be seriously depressed because of the possibility of death which they faced, were noted to be unexpectedly content and happy. It quickly became apparent that this drug had anti-depressive properties, and in 1958 it became one of the group of antidepressants known as monoamine oxidase inhibitors (MAOIs) This helped establish the relationship between psychiatric disorder and brain chemistry. Around the same time, another antidepressant, imipramine (Tofranil), was synthesised, and in 1957 it became the first tricyclic antidepressant (TCA) in medical use. For several decades these antidepressant groups dominated the treatment of depressive illness.

Before the discovery of antidepressants, Italian neurologist Ugo Cerletti and his assistant, Lucio Bini, discovered electroconvulsive therapy (ECT). It was first used in 1938, on a patient diagnosed with schizophrenia who had delusions and hallucinations. The outcome was positive and thus was born one of the most controversial treatments in psychiatry.

Another early landmark was the finding by John Cade, an Australian working in Melbourne, that lithium had a role in treating mania. In 1954 Mogens Schou, a Danish psychiatrist, demonstrated that it had a role in preventing relapses in bipolar disorder (then called manic depression). Its use was still limited until 1970, when the US Food and Drugs Administration (FDA) finally allowed for the use of lithium in the treatment of acute mania and, in 1975, in preventing manic relapses. Thereafter it became the drug of choice for the prevention of relapse in bipolar disorder, reducing the number of hospitalisations. It continues to be the mood stabiliser with the best evidence base. It has also become important in the management of treatment-resistant depression.

The first effective treatment for schizophrenia was chlorpromazine, which was first used by a French naval surgeon post-operatively. He noticed that the drug had a calming effect and wondered if it might help psychiatric patients. In 1952, two French psychiatrists, Jean Delay and Paul Deniker, used the drug to treat their patients and found that it had a beneficial effect. This was the first antipsychotic drug to be used in psychiatry. The beneficial effects of these drugs cannot be overstated. Before their introduction 70% of those with a diagnosis of schizophrenia were confined to hospital for many years, and often permanently. Today, only 5% of those with schizophrenia require lengthy periods in hospital, and even then the stay is counted in months rather than years.

Clozapine was another revolutionary drug in the treatment of schizophrenia, developed in the 1990s for those with treatment-resistant disorder or with 'negative' symptoms of schizophrenia, such as social withdrawal and poor motivation. These features became the hallmark of chronic illness. This medication is superior to older drugs like chlorpromazine in treating negative symptoms of schizophrenia.

These milestones provided more effective treatments for those with severe mental illness and facilitated the closure of large 'asylums' for those with mental illnesses that were hitherto untreatable.

Non-pharmacological therapies also emerged in the 1960s. Prior to this, the main 'talking therapy' was Freudian psychoanalysis, a very long-term therapy associated with the rich and famous in Hollywood. Talking therapy was non-existent for the majority of those in psychiatric hospitals. This changed with the growth of behaviour therapy, developed in the 1950s by Joseph Wolpe, a South African psychiatrist working in Virginia, US. He was strongly influenced by his work in treating soldiers for post-traumatic stress disorder (PTSD). He was initially a supporter of Freudian psycho-analysis, but when he found this to be unsuccessful in treating his patients, he sought to develop other approaches. He turned to behaviourism as a theoretical model, and developed a technique called systematic desensitisation. Behaviour therapy was widely practised in the 1970s and 80s.

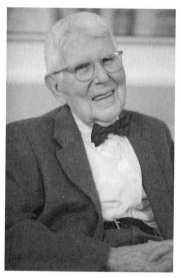

Portrait of Aaron T. Beck.

In 1967 Aaron Beck, a psychologist at the University of Pennsylvania, developed a time-limited talking therapy that was accessible to large numbers of people. Cognitive therapy, as it came to be called, focused not on the past but on the person's current thinking, and on the false assumptions in thinking that the patient makes that reinforce illness. By incorporating elements of behavioural techniques it became known as cognitive behavioural therapy (CBT). This therapy was and remains very helpful in treating conditions such as obsessive-compulsive disorder (OCD), mild depression, and anxiety. Alongside medication, the combination optimises treatment for depression and anxiety, and also for some psychotic symptoms such as chronic hallucinations. It is widely available, and is the approach now most commonly used by clinical psychologists.

LEGISLATIVE CHANGES

The law governing the treatment of those with mental illness obviously differs from country to country and time to time. In this book, the focus is on Irish law. In Ireland, as in all countries, treatment is now normally voluntarily sought. For those requiring, but refusing, treatment, when they pose a risk to the safety of themselves or others, there are legal protections in place to allow them to be detained against their will. Until 2001 this was governed by the Mental Treatment Act 1945. Its flaws made it unfit for purpose and it was replaced by the Mental Health Act 2001, which is the law governing current practice (see Chapter 13).

DEFINING MENTAL ILLNESS AND MENTAL HEALTH

Severe mental illness or 'insanity' has been recognised for centuries. Yet arriving at a definition that captures the breadth of the conditions we now see in modern psychiatric practice, from phobias and eating disorders to unexplained physical symptoms and schizophrenia, is a conceptual challenge. There is no single all-embracing definition of mental disorder (also referred to as mental illness) that clearly delineates disorder from normality or mental illness from mental health. However, attempts have been made to provide such a definition, and the profession most frequently looks to the World Health Organisation (WHO) for this.

WHO definition of mental disorder and mental health

> **Mental disorders** comprise a broad range of problems, with different symptoms. They are generally characterised by some combination of disturbed thoughts, emotions, behaviour and relationships with others.
> **Mental health** is a state of well-being in which an individual can realise their own potential, cope with the normal stresses of life, work productively and make a contribution to the community.

We should note two things about the WHO definition. First, the conditions are referred to as 'problems'; second, an illness emerges from some *combination* of symptoms emerging from these problems. Consider a person who is grieving following the death of a loved one. That person will likely be described as having a 'problem'. They will usually show disturbed emotions (sadness, pining) and possibly disturbed thoughts (reminiscing about the past with the person, feeling guilty that they should have done more). Their behaviour may change as they withdraw from meeting others in an attempt to avoid the pain of being asked about their loss. Moreover, for most who experience a bereavement, these features are present for a prolonged period of time, such as several months after the event. Based on this definition, many who experience grief would be classified as being mentally ill. However, this grief response is in fact perfectly normal and healthy. This simple example illustrates how difficult it is to separate the sadness and troubles of life from mental illness, and thereby how difficult it is to formulate an adequate definition of mental illness.

There is an obverse problem with the WHO definition of mental health. It can lead to a diagnosis of mental illness in cases of normal, healthy people going through trying times. What if a person doesn't realise their potential through an innate lack of ambition? Are they mentally unhealthy? Do they suffer from a disorder? Is making a contribution to society too high a bar to expect an unemployed person living in social housing to meet? Are they mentally disordered for not meeting it? Why should the extent of a person's contribution to society be a measure of their mental well-being? These questions demonstrate the potential problems with the WHO definition of mental health, which seems to be closely bound up with social measures. These are questions for the WHO and those interested in the boundary between mental illness/disorder and mental health to consider.

THE ICD AND DSM: WHAT ARE THEY?

The WHO is not alone in attempting to formulate a definition of mental illness. The American Psychiatric Association (APA) has also concerned itself with defining and describing psychiatric conditions. Both organisations' approach is to list the disorders currently recognised as being psychiatric, and to describe the symptoms and their duration in each condition. These descriptions are contained in two manuals that are regularly updated. The WHO produces the *International Classification of Diseases* (ICD), currently in its 10th edition (ICD-10, 1994), and the APA publishes the *Diagnostic and Statistical Manual* (DSM), now in its 5th edition (DSM-5, 2013). Copies of both are available online and both, but especially the DSM, are often referred to as 'the Bible of psychiatry'. I disagree with the assessment, as I think that both manuals have serious flaws, although there have been benefits also, most particularly the improvement in the reliability of diagnoses between specialists.

The thinking behind both of these classifications is that the symptoms of psychiatric conditions, like medical disorders, should be clearly specified to allow accurate diagnoses to be made. In this way there should be no uncertainty about the diagnosis, whether a patient is seen in Cork, Chicago or Cairo. This is termed 'reliability' in medical jargon. It was an attempt to overcome the charge that 'doctors differ and patients die' – in other words that two doctors might diagnose the same patient differently and, in consequence, the patient would suffer. In psychiatry, the drive towards reliability came about partly because of a study that found that the symptoms necessary to make a diagnosis of bipolar disorder differed as between the UK and the US. The investigation, known as the UK-US Diagnostic Study, found that bipolar disorder was diagnosed more frequently in Britain than in the US, whereas in the latter, schizophrenia was more frequent. This was not simply because there were real differences between the two jurisdictions but because the same symptoms were regarded differently in each country. Since the first DSM in 1952, and the first ICD to include psychiatric disorders, ICD-6 (1947), the two glossaries have continued to differ in the list of specific psychiatric disorders as well as in their diagnostic features.

With the publication of DSM-5 in 2013 and the upcoming release of ICD-11 in 2021, it was hoped to bring the two closer together. Attempts at alignment have improved, but it has not yet been fully achieved.

In general medicine, diagnosis is not based just on the obvious symptoms, such as those the patient would complain of. Diagnosis is also based on various blood tests and radiological tests, and perhaps other investigations such as biopsies. However, this extended diagnosis, known as 'biological investigation', is not possible in psychiatry, and despite the ambition that we would have biological investigations available early in the 21st century, this has not come about. This is likely due to the challenges that working with a complex organ like the brain poses. Psychiatrists still have to rely exclusively on only two sources of evidence:

first, the symptoms that the patient describes, and, second, the symptoms that others identify in the patient. In other words, the patient's psychiatric and medical history is the cornerstone of making a psychiatric diagnosis. The subjective nature of psychiatric history-taking is a continuing cause for concern. In addition, when a mental health professional makes an enquiry about the patient's past, they are reliant on the patient's memory, which is not always reliable (this is known as recall bias).

The symptoms that are used to make a diagnosis are referred to the diagnostic criteria. An example of these is shown in Chapter 3, for both ICD-10 and DSM-5.

CONTROVERSIES IN PSYCHIATRY

Psychiatry, like any other branch of medicine, is rife with vigorous internal debates, many of which have no merit. Yet debate should not be frowned upon: it is through such discussion and even disagreement that scientific and medical progress is made. However, psychiatry is also a site of some more extreme controversies, and, indeed, there are some people, who describe themselves as anti-psychiatry, who think that the entire specialty is illegitimate. This is a unique challenge faced by psychiatry: there are no anti-surgery groups or anti-pathology groups!

There are four broad critiques of psychiatry as a specialty:

Criticisms of Psychiatry

1. Mental illness does not exist.
2. The origins of mental illness are social and psychological, not biological.
3. The origins of mental illness are multiple, but there is too much emphasis on the biological.
4. Mental illness is multifactorial but it is over-diagnosed.

Firstly, there are those who do not accept that mental illness exists at all. Thomas Szasz, who wrote the influential book *The Myth of Mental Illness* (1961), is the name most strongly associated with this view. He argued that there can be no illness of the mind, and so the term 'mental illness' is oxymoronic. He believed that psychiatry was akin to alchemy and that it offended the idea of personal liberty. Instead of 'treating' deviation using medication, people, he argued, should be taught personal responsibility. Opponents of this view point to the positive role medication has played in closing psychiatric hospitals. In terms of responsibility his view seems harsh and judgemental. How would one deal with those who commit offences when mentally ill – should they therefore be sent to prison rather than to hospital?

In his book *The Divided Self* (1965) R. D. Laing saw the oppression of the family as the main contributor to mental illness, and he supported ideas such as the 'double-bind hypothesis' of schizophrenia, a concept later disproven. He viewed schizophrenia as '*a special strategy that a person invents in order to live in an unliveable situation*'. His work was based on individual case studies rather than large group studies and has not stood the test of time.

A third view accepts that mental illness has biological as well as psychological and social origins, but argues that there has been an over-emphasis on the biological elements. The Critical Psychiatry Group, formed in the UK in 1999, is particularly exercised by the necessity for diagnosis and by the use of medication. The group has concerns about the link between psychiatrists and pharma. The organisation, whose co-chair is Professor Joanna Moncrieff, has expressed concern about the use of medications such as antidepressants, mood stabilisers and antipsychotic agents, and it is also critical of psychiatric diagnosis because of its use in detaining people under the mental health legislation. The members of the Critical Psychiatry Group believe that psychiatrists are acting as agents of social control.

A fourth view accepts that mental illness exists, and accepts that the origins are biological, psychological or social. Proponents of this view differ from those in the third group in believing that diagnosis is appropriate since this aids in deciding on treatment. They prescribe medication but believe that mental illness is over-diagnosed due to a blurring of the boundary between normality and illness (Horwitz and Wakefield, 2007). This is a consequence of the approach to diagnosis in the DSM in particular, and to a lesser extent in the ICD, which has resulted in an excessive use of both pharmacological and psychological interventions (Casey, 2016; Francis, 2009) for what are normal responses to life situations. This is termed the 'medicalisation of everyday life', and it applies more to depression and other common disorders than to psychoses such as bipolar disorder or schizophrenia.

For a more detailed exploration of the medicalisation of everyday life, see *Our Necessary Shadow* by my colleague Professor Tom Burns (2013).

ARE DIAGNOSES NECESSARY?

One of the central points made by the first three anti-psychiatry schools relates to the role of diagnosis. They note that psychiatric diagnosis is not based on any physical or biological measures, and also point out that they are stigmatising and that their application leads to social control of those so labelled. (Furthermore, those in the first group would add that if mental illness does not exist then of course it can't be diagnosed.) They argue on these grounds that psychiatric diagnosis is, as such, illegitimate.

Yet, for time immemorial, mental illness has been recognised. Hippocrates identified it and developed his humoral theory. It is recognised in the Bible and in the Koran. Of course it was not called mental illness then, but was attributed to other factors such as demonic possession and the lunar cycle, hence the term 'lunacy'. Regardless of how it was described or explained, it was acknowledged as real.

Over time, our understanding of mental illness has improved, and we have seen a complementary development of terminology to reflect what were believed to be disease processes, such as 'dementia praecox'. This term, which literally translates as 'early dementia', was once the term for schizophrenia that resulted in changes so grave in the person's ability to function that psychiatric institutions were founded to house the sufferers. These institutions became less necessary as more and better antipsychotic agents were developed.

The central argument against such labels as schizophrenia, panic disorder and so on is that they stigmatise and dehumanise people. The other argument is that a single label is grossly insufficient when trying to explain the complexity of some of the emotions and experiences that those with mental illness have to contend with.

Some also point out that there is often little diagnostic agreement when two different psychiatrists see the same patient. This phenomenon is known as the *low reliability* of psychiatric diagnosis. So as to standardise diagnosis, specific diagnostic criteria have been developed for both the ICD and DSM systems.

One of the basic reasons for making a diagnosis is so that people who have similar symptoms can be studied as a group. This would allow us to identify attributes that increase the risk of the illness and would enable possible treatments to be tested in similar groups. By contrast, if every individual with symptoms were regarded as different from every other, how could treatments be tried and tested? How could we identify who was vulnerable if the common features were not identified?

The proponenets of the third view are right that diagnoses of mental illness can stigmatise patients. However, patients themselves like to know what diagnosis they have, whether in medicine or psychiatry. So, in the same way that physicians and surgeons will tell patients that they have coronary artery disease or appendicitis, a psychiatrist will also tell patients that they have generalised anxiety or a depressive episode.

People like and value a diagnostic label. With this information to hand they can be provided with treatments that have been shown to be beneficial in these specific diagnoses and will be advised of likely side effects. Patients themselves can carry out their own personal research online into what is known about the condition and will therefore feel empowered. None of this would be possible if we did not use diagnostic labels. Human beings themselves think in categorical terms like age (above or below 65), employment, marital status and so on. Offering a diagnostic label is in tune with the categorical way of thinking that is part of the human psyche and that allows us to make sense of our world. Of course, it is true that diagnoses of mental illnesses can be stigmatising for sufferers, as the proponents of the third view note: but the problem here does not lie with psychiatrists for diagnosing the illnesses, but with society for stigmatising those with mental illness. Consider an imaginary parallel case: if people with diabetes were stigmatised, the fault here would lie, not with the doctors diagnosing diabetes, but with society for stigmatising those with diabetes. It would still be appropriate for doctors to diagnose diabetes when that was the medically correct diagnosis. Similarly in psychiatry, it is important for psychiatrists to make the psychiatrically correct diagnosis. Stigmatisation of mental illness remains a huge problem, however, and so the work done by celebrities such as Princes William and Harry, comedian Russell Brand, footballer Paul McGrath and many others like them is hugely important and laudable.

ARE DIAGNOSES BEING INVENTED? THE VALIDITY PROBLEM

Notwithstanding the benefits of and necessity for diagnosis, there is a problem with the number of new disorders that have been added to the psychiatric terminology over the years. The question is, are these real disorders or are they simplistic terms applied in an ad hoc manner? What about reactive attachment disorder or parental alienation or sex addiction? Are these real disorders or simply behaviours that are part of the human condition that stem from social problems or bad habits? Why should psychiatry take these on board as disorders when they are generated by the frailties of human life? Whether these conditions, that now have labels, are real in the sense of existing in the way that diabetes or arthritis or schizophrenia exist, is open to question.

An important term in psychiatry is *validity*. Validity here is defined as the fact that a constellation of symptoms, or an entity, described as a disorder, actually merits this description. For the entity to be a valid psychiatric disorder it must be shown to have (a) a known cause (aetiology), (b) identifying symptoms, (c) a response to treatment and (d) a predictable course in the future (Kendall and Jablensky, 2003). Unfortunately, many of the conditions identified in DSM and ICD do not meet these requirements, which apply to most of the labels associated with personality disorder.

Both the ICD and DSM are updated every decade or even more frequently. DSM was updated in 2013 and ICD-11 is currently in the process of being developed – it is due to become operational in 2021. Taking DSM as an example of the expansion of psychiatric diagnoses, the first edition in 1952 named 106 disorders, the fourth edition (DSM-IV) in 1994 had 279, and DSM-5 in 2013 had 297. Both DSM and ICD have added new categories and removed some categories that had previously existed. For example, the diagnoses 'reactive depression' and 'Asperger's syndrome' have been removed, but sex addiction, reactive attachment disorder, caffeine intoxication, parental alienation syndrome, gaming disorder, to name but a few, have been added. The possibility that some of these new additions will later be recognised as problems of living rather than psychiatric diagnosis is very real, as they will fall short of the requirements for a valid disorder listed above.

BIBLIOGRAPHY

American Psychiatric Association: *Diagnostic and Statistical Manual of Mental Disorders*, 5th Edition. Washington, DC: American Psychiatric Association. 2013.

Burns, T. *Our Necessary Shadow: The Nature and Meaning of Psychiatry*. London: Penguin. 2013.

Casey, P., and Strain, J. 'Borderline Between Normal and Pathological Responses'. *Trauma and Stressor-related Disorders: A Handbook for Clinicians*. Washington, DC: American Psychiatric Publishing. 2016.

Frances, Allen. 'Whither DSM-V?' *British Journal of Psychiatry*. 195. 391–92. 2009

Horwitz, A., and Wakefield, J. *The Loss of Sadness: How Psychiatry Transformed Normal Sorrow into Depressive Disorder*. New York, NY: Oxford University Press. 2007.

Kelly, B. *Hearing Voices: The History of Psychiatry in Ireland*. Dublin: Irish Academic Press. 2019.

Kendall, R. and Jablensky, A. Distinguishing between the validity and utility of psychiatric diagnoses. *American Journal of Psychiatry*. 160: 2–12. 2003.

Laing, R.D. *The Divided Self: An Existential Study in Sanity and Madness*. London: Penguin Modern Classics. 1965.

Szasz, T. *The Myth of Mental Illness: Foundations of a Theory of Personal Conduct*. New York, NY: Harper and Row. 1961.

World Health Organisation. *International Classification of Diseases*, 11th ed. Geneva: World Health Organisation. 2019.

2

Organisation of the Psychiatric Services

The focus of the treatment of those with mental illness was exclusively hospital-based from the 19th century onwards. Prior to that, there had been some private treatment facilities in Ireland and Europe, but the early 1800s saw the emergence of psychiatric hospitals for the poor who were mentally ill. These hospitals were behind high walls, usually located deep in the countryside, and the period of hospitalisation usually lasted many years, if not a lifetime. During the late 1800s and into the early 20th century the numbers admitted to such hospitals increased dramatically and they became greatly overcrowded with very few therapeutic facilities. There was very little treatment available apart from basic day-to-day care, and large numbers of people never left them. Between the 1800s, when asylums were first built, until the late 1950s, the number of admissions climbed, peaking in the 1950s, when Ireland had the highest known rate of psychiatric bed occupancy in Europe (Brennan, 2014). In 1963 19,801 people were institutionalised in Irish psychiatric hospitals; by 2003 this number had fallen to 3,658 (Kelly, 2017).

Since then, breakthroughs in drug treatments and the development of accessible psychological interventions such as behaviour therapy and then cognitive therapy from the 1960s revolutionised psychiatric practice. People heretofore confined to psychiatric institutions, behind high walls, could now be discharged home. Gradually the walls of enclosure came tumbling down and modern psychiatry was born.

CHANGING ATTITUDES AND SERVICE DEVELOPMENT

The closure of mental hospitals was gradual in some countries (such as Ireland and Britain), but in others it was more rapid. Trieste in Italy was notable for the very dramatic manner of the change from institutional to community care. Between 1971 and 1977 all the psychiatric institutions there were closed. Patients were sent back into the community, with limited facilities. This was hailed by supporters of Franco Basaglia, the psychiatrist who spearheaded this revolution, as a momentous achievement, and by others as ideologically driven, chaotic and a 'disaster'.

In Ireland our mental health policy was driven by a document called *Planning for the Future* (1984). This established a comprehensive and community-focused policy for those with mental illness and, increasingly, treatment was delivered in community-based outpatient clinics, with close GP liaison. In 2006 this policy was updated in a document called *A Vision for Change*, which remains the blueprint for the delivery of psychiatric services in Ireland.

A Vision for Change recommends that the population should be divided into geographic areas, more commonly referred to as 'psychiatric sectors', each with between 25,000 and 30,000 people. Each sector has a consultant, or sometimes two, who delivers a multidisciplinary service that includes not just a consultant and junior doctors but also clinical psychologists, psychiatric social workers, occupational therapists, counsellors and community mental health nurses. Inpatient beds are now almost all in general hospitals. Patient advocates are available for any patient who requests them, to speak on their behalf in their dealings with members of the multidisciplinary team and other agencies.

There is also a focus on rehabilitation, and consultants in this specialism of psychiatry have been appointed throughout the country to help those who have been hospitalised for prolonged periods to retrain and re-enter the workforce subsequent to discharge. It is important to understand that only a minority of patients need this, since most make a good recovery, and very few require long-term inpatient treatment.

In addition, *A Vision for Change* emphasised the necessity for a close relationship between patients (also referred to as 'service users'), carers, the treating teams and other stakeholders, such as housing agencies. There is a recognition of the link between social exclusion and mental illness, and the emphasis in *A Vision for Change* is on establishing and promoting community-based protective factors such as housing, occupation and social supports. These protections enhance patients' resilience against relapses.

THE PROBLEM WITH BEDS

A Vision for Change recommends that one community mental health team should be provided per 50,000 people, with two consultant psychiatrists per team. It also says that there should be 50 inpatient beds per 300,000 people. The breakdown of beds per capita is further specified, too: the document says that within each of these 30,000-person groups, there should be 35 beds for the general adult mental health services for those aged 18–64, eight for mental health services for those over 65, five for people with learning disability, and two for those with eating disorders. Shamefully, these recommendations are woefully inadequate. Our inpatient bed numbers are the third lowest in the EU according to Eurostat data, ahead of only Cyprus and Italy. Thus we have moved from having had the highest number of inpatients until the 1960s, to having the third lowest number of inpatient beds in the EU. Previously the human rights issues in psychiatry concerned over-reliance on custodial care, but now the issue is the right of access to appropriate inpatient care when needed. This is indeed a full swing of the treatment pendulum.

An area that is seldom discussed by stakeholders and by the media is the problem of prisoners with mental illness. Some prison inmates are there because of offending behaviour in the context of untreated mental illness. Prison is unhelpful and even damaging to this group, who require treatment, not punishment. Indeed, the number of mentally ill offenders increased following the closure of our mental hospitals. Prisoners in this situation should be referred to and treated by the forensic psychiatric service, but this has failed to keep pace with demand. There are between 25 and 30 prisoners waiting for beds in the Central Mental Hospital

(CMH) at any one time. The CMH is our only hospital for those who are charged with or guilty of serious crime associated with mental illness. However, things in this respect are improving: in early 2021 the CMH is to relocate from Dunrum to Portrane, where it will have 130 medium and high secure beds, 30 low secure beds and 10 beds for children and adolescents This marks a substantial increase in capacity, but this new hospital will still have a substantially lower treatment capacity than other similar hospitals in Europe (Kelly, 2019).

A persistent problem in Irish mental health care is that where you live affects how accessible psychiatric services and inpatient beds are. This is particularly a problem if a person is homeless and has no fixed address. Services use different criteria for admitting a homeless person. For example, one will accept for admission a patient who presents to that hospital, but others will refuse and refer the patient to the hospital closest to their last known address, or to a hospital where they had previously been a patient. The homeless person then becomes the unfortunate victim of bargaining, as the hospitals bicker over who has to admit them. The problem, however, is not confined to the homeless. If a patient known to a particular service, perhaps for many years, moves to an area covered by a different team, that person's care will then be transferred. This may be appropriate for a person who has high demands and who has frequent involvement with community nurses, day hospitals and so on. However, for the person who is well and simply requires the occasional check-up every few months, this can be very disruptive to the continuity of care. In practice, unfortunately, there is little or no flexibility in this. Psychiatry truly does enshrine the Eircode in its practices in an inordinately inflexible manner, even to the point that a consultant not wishing to transfer a person's care for very good clinical reasons will be unable to access any ancillary facilities, such as community nurse follow-up, for that person. I have personal experience of that.

In addition to inpatient beds, there are day hospitals, where those who are not ill enough to be inpatients, but who require more input than out-patient clinics can provide, can attend. Talking therapies are commonly used alongside drug treatments in these settings. Attendance at the day hospital is usually brief: seldom more than a few hours per week for a few weeks.

Home care teams also operate out of the day hospitals. These teams provide nursing care to those being treated in the setting of their own home. They do not provide full day care, as some assume, but have a visiting and monitoring role, particularly at weekends, for those being treated at home. This may occur if the person refuses inpatient care and for some reason cannot be certified (see p.240), or if they have limited access to a day hospital.

HOW ARE THE PSYCHIATRIC SERVICES ACCESSED?

The most common route to accessing psychiatric services is by referral from a person's GP to the multidisciplinary team that covers the geographic area in which the person lives (the 'catchment' area or sector). The person will be evaluated by a member of that team and then seen by the consultant. A treatment plan will be developed and appropriate follow-up arranged. This may be to the team's outpatient clinic, to its day hospital or, if the person is ill enough, to its inpatient unit. Those wishing to avail of private care can be referred by their GP to any private psychiatrist.

The second way of accessing psychiatric care is to attend the emergency department for evaluation. This is more common in cases where the problem is acute. There will be an initial assessment by one of the general emergency department doctors, who will then refer the person to the psychiatrist on call. This will be a junior doctor who will discuss the person with the duty consultant; after this, a follow-up with the appropriate psychiatric team will be arranged.

Any hospital doctor can refer a person to a psychiatrist. Physicians and surgeons commonly do so while people are being treated by them as inpatients for a separate physical complaint, but outpatients who have mental health problems may also be referred, usually to one of the in-house psychiatrists.

THE MULTIDISCIPLINARY TEAM

This team of mental health professionals that is recommended by *A Vision for Change* is referred to as the multidisciplinary team (MDT) (see page 28).

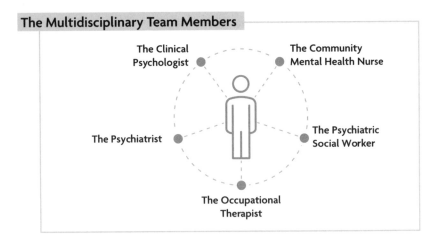

The Multidisciplinary Team Members

- The Clinical Psychologist
- The Community Mental Health Nurse
- The Psychiatrist
- The Psychiatric Social Worker
- The Occupational Therapist

Teams that are well resourced may additionally have music or art therapists, lifestyle coaches, family and relationship therapists and counsellors.

HAS *A VISION FOR CHANGE* BEEN A SUCCESS?

The aspirations of *A Vision for Change* were welcomed by the profession. The obvious question now is, 'Have the goals of *A Vision for Change* been realised?' The answer is no. Indeed, we have fallen short of meeting a great number of its goals. Some of these relate to the actual number of available mental health professionals, while others relate to the areas of specialist expertise, and yet others to work practices and availability of essential therapies.

1. Not all of the multidisciplinary teams have the full compliment of disciplines.

2. Consultant numbers are below the numbers recommended in *all* specialties, and particularly in child and adolescent psychiatry. There is also a shortage of psychiatric nurses countrywide.

3. There is a move towards having two consultants on each team, but this is not universal and, where there are two, they appear to operate separately, with little flexibility in relation to patient care. Sometimes one does inpatient work while the other is based in the community. Sometimes the area is split geographically

between each. Thus, an individual with a mental health problem living in a particular geographic area will only be able to attend the consultant in that particular sector. If there are conflicts with the patient, transfer of care to a different consultant is difficult.

4. *A Vision for Change* recommended a number of 'crisis houses' with 10 places per 300,000 people, four intensive care units with 30 beds each, eight high-support residences, and 10 places per 100,000 people for early intervention assessment. This would focus on those with risk factors for schizophrenia or possibly early symptoms of the condition. Most of these additional services have not been realised.

5. Specific psychiatric disorders require additional expertise over and above the usual competencies that all consultant psychiatrists possess. In this regard sector teams often lack the totality of the skill mix required to treat the range of disorders seen in clinical practice. In particular, the treatment of eating disorders and of personality disorders is limited.

6. In some specific subspecialties there are staff shortages – this is particularly a problem in early intervention services for those who may have emerging severe mental illness, in services for the homeless, and in perinatal psychiatry, to name but a few.

7. Vitally important therapies such as dialectical behaviour therapy, for the treatment of those who repeatedly self-harm, are sporadic and not available in many mental health sectors.

8. As a consequence of staff shortages there are long waiting lists, particularly in child psychiatry and psychology.

OUTPATIENT SERVICES

Most of those referred to psychiatrists by their GPs or by other doctors such as physicians and surgeons will never need to be admitted to hospital. Many will be able to continue working, although some may require temporary sick leave if their illness is impacting on their day-to-day functioning. Only those who are acutely psychotic (due to schizophrenia or bipolar disorder) or suicidal will require admission.

The outpatient clinics may be held in local health centres or in general hospital outpatient departments. Those seeing psychologists, social workers, or other mental health professionals will also do this in the outpatient clinic or health centre. Community psychiatric nurses visit people in their homes. It is they who also run clinics specifically for those taking the drug clozapine, since this requires close monitoring of blood levels and of the actual composition of the blood itself due to the side effects of this treatment.

THE ROLE OF THE GENERAL PRACTITIONER

The GP plays a large role in making the initial referral to a psychiatrist, although hospital-based doctors, such as neurologists, gastroenterologists etc., increasingly make referrals as well. The majority of people with mental health problems do not need to see a psychiatrist. Treatment is offered mainly by GPs. Alongside this, psychological services, to which GPs now have direct access, have been established. This has led to the development of the Counselling in Primary Care Service (CIPC). This is a counselling service for those with mild-to-moderate psychological difficulties, and it provides up to eight counselling sessions by a professionally qualified counsellor or psychologist. It is available to medical card holders over the age of 18. Details about CIPC can be found on the HSE website, which provides a wealth of information on this service and the range of conditions for which it offers help.

The GP also plays a crucial role in the certification of patients who *require* compulsory admission under the Mental Health Act 2000. This is discussed further in Chapter 14.

BIBLIOGRAPHY

Brennan, D. *Irish Insanity: 1800–2000* (Routledge Advances in Sociology). London: Routledge. 2014.

Expert Group of Mental Health Policy. *A Vision for Change.* Dublin: Stationery Office. 2006.

Kelly, B. 'Mental Health Services in Ireland'. *Mental health in Ireland.* Dublin: Liffey Press. 2017

Kelly, B. 'Ireland must tackle its mental health deficit disorder'. *The Irish Times.* 10 December 2019.

Shorter, E. *A History of Psychiatry: From the Era of the Asylum to the Age of Prozac.* 2nd edition. London: Wiley. 1998.

Study Group on the Development of the Psychiatric Services. *The Psychiatric Services. – Planning for the Future.* Dublin: Stationery Office. 1984.

USEFUL RESOURCES

www.hse.ie mental health services (for Counselling in Primary Care Information) or https://www.hse.ie/eng/services/list/4/mental-health-services/counsellingpc/

THE LIVED EXPERIENCE

Setting up a support group – by service users for service users

---

The Phrenz Group Galway is a support group for people enduring schizophrenia and other mental health issues. We meet in the day centre, Danesfield, Sea Road, Galway, on Thursday evenings.

A nurse, M, from the Psychiatric Unit in Galway, asked a service user would he like to set up and organise a group for people who endured schizophrenia in the Galway city area 25 years ago. With the help of family carers he waited in a room for three months every week until people came to know of the group's meetings. At that time there were far more women than men coming to the meetings. Over the years this has changed, and now mostly men attend. We have moved to many different venues over the years. The day centre at Danesfield has been our home for 15 years now.

The Phrenz Group Galway offers support and a way to deal with social isolation. Simply being labelled with schizophrenia diagnoses can cause huge stigma to members and personal withdrawal from society may occur. Indeed, many older members see the Phrenz Group as a social group as well as a support group

The Phrenz Group Galway have no intention of giving advice to members. We offer support. Some new members do not understand this. They come in with their difficulties and want answers. They get very disillusioned with this policy of offering no advice and we never see them again. We will signpost members towards medical assistance, social welfare professionals and organisations for work etc. Members have to work through their difficulties. We provide empathy to members enduring difficulties

The highlight of the year in the Phrenz Group is going on a holiday with members. We usually go to Westport and stay in the Castlecourt Hotel for three days. In 2020, due to the Covid-19 crisis, we obtained no funding from Shine, the Lottery or public fundraising for the holiday. However, the group went on holiday in September when the lockdown was lifted.

The members paid for this holiday. I am very proud that the members took this action with no support. We cannot moan if there is a window of opportunity. The holiday was a great success. The members rigidly stuck by the Covid-19 restrictions – but still enjoyed themselves.

It was with regret that we no longer have our facilitator, TN, this year. She is now working in the mental health recovery college Galway and is too busy to commit to us. Usually a facilitator organises and guides the group meeting. The facilitator liaises with and is paid by Shine West.

We in The Phrenz Group do not waste our members' time. The facilitator is required to work an orderly meeting. Great emphasis is placed on the members helping one another. We are all allowed and requested to talk on our week and any challenges we may have. Some members will not say a word – but they still come for support. We have a cup of tea before the meeting, not after, as is more normal. We find this encourages fun and less energy is needed when we go in to the meeting proper.

At the meeting we rarely talk about medication. We insist that members always take their medication. There is a plethora of medication nowadays and only doctors are qualified to advise on medication. However, we constantly ask members to relate their medication difficulties to doctors. As many members endure side effects of medication, we, with our experience, are able to help with these side effects.

We have done many training courses over the years and have educated ourselves in cooking, art, pottery and photography.

We have many achievements. Most of our members were cigarette smokers. There are now only two members who smoke. Members are proud of the fact that there has been only a handful of hospital readmissions in the 25 years since the group came into existence. This shows that the group works and that members take their own healthcare seriously.

Challenges remain. We need new members. We are in danger of becoming too old, with no young people to take over. The Covid-19 crisis necessitates different ways of holding meetings. In 2020 there were no meetings of The Phrenz Group. Shine would not allow them due to the pandemic.

The Phrenz Group was a huge help in providing a new wave of approaches for mental health services in Galway over the years, including drop-in centres. They also support the Recovery College in NUIG. There is also Mr Waffle café, a meeting place for service users. This will be up and running after the Covid-19 crisis is over.

I began working with the Galway Phrenz group fours ago, as part of Shine's peer support groups, run around the country. Having trained as a facilitator with Shine a few years previously, I was delighted to get this post. This involved facilitating a peer support group, which met once a week for about two hours. It was a social space also, where members of the group shared their concerns, struggles and experiences with medication, provided effective support for each other and had good fun. The group is well established for many years in Galway. Some of the members were founding members of the group and had been involved in other initiatives of providing valuable service user input in making the mental health services more recovery focused, with varying degrees of success over the past 25 years.

From the very beginning, the group made me feel very welcome, and I was both impressed and humbled by the generosity and mutual support that was available in the group. This support extended beyond the group sessions, with members providing practical support for each other, e.g. accompanying someone on a visit to the doctor, or helping someone to negotiate with the City Council for repairs to boilers or replacing a cooker. My time with the group has been one of the most fulfilling jobs of my career. It has shown me the value of peer support among people with mental health challenges, and the need for the HSE to support such groups.

Social isolation – through the eyes of a service user ...

Musings on the aforementioned topic:

Well! ... Well! ... Well! The theme is social isolation.

I know it only too well. The doctor said to me: 'I think you are a bit of a loner!' In any kind of relationship, I tend to come in last, an also-ran, the loser in the race! What can I say?

Looking back, I remember a time when the straitjacket was still on the table and the male nurse had just left the room and was walking down the corridor. While that time is long gone, I still recall the feelings of despair, those days of despair which turned into nights, where my only companions were my own negative thoughts.

As I mused on the past, the long, lonely night stretched ahead into a broken dawn and I knew there would be little sleep. I also knew that the early morning depression never seemed to live up to or measure up to, the progress of the night before.

I woke with a start, a bad dream! It must have been that blasted chicken tikka masala from the night before. Remind me not to eat take-away food again. It is playing havoc with my digestive system, not to mention my diabetes. I knew it was going to be a Bad Day ahead.

I packed a few belongings into an overnight bag, pyjamas, toi-letries, tablets, a few changes of clothes and a few of my beloved books. I knew I didn't really want to go into hospital for a stint but I also knew I probably had little choice and I thought that it might do me good anyway to meet up with other people there. So I went without a fuss.

I spent about a week in the hospital. It was a bit of a disappointment. I had to stay on my own most of the time and could not go within two metres of anyone else. Most of the staff went around in PPE and masks and gloves. Other patients were also restricted and forced to wear masks and gloves to avoid the Covid-19 virus.

I felt I had to get out of there. In there, I felt even more socially isolated than before and I feared that I might pick up the virus if I was there for much longer. Finally, one morning the doctor called in to my room and told me I was being released. Great, I thought, I would be able to return to my humble apartment which, while lonely, would still give me independence. The doctor also told me that the virus restrictions were to be eased shortly so I would have more freedom to go out and about and meet friends and acquaintances.

To celebrate, I rang Boutros Boutros, my best friend, to share the good news. Life is not so bad after all.

I remembered the advice given by a member of SEE CHANGE: 'Do not give interviews on days when you are not at your best'.

This was one of those days, so I rang my PA and asked her to cancel all my appointments for the day. You don't have any appointments today, she said. So I thanked her and took my tablets for the day instead.

I could have been something or someone, I thought, if only the chips had fallen in my favour. Another broken dream, I mused. Another wasted Nowhere! Another wasted Nothingness! To complete a full circle of nihilism ... Nowhere meets Nothingness on the way back! Anyway, enough of this foolish meandering, I thought. It won't get you nowhere, I chided myself, and there were practical matters to which I needed to attend.

After breakfast consisting of Weetabix with milk and some fruit and a yogurt, I rang my PA again. This time she said she was not my PA, never was and never will be. If I didn't get off the phone and stop stalking her, she said, she would call the guards. Later that morning, I had a visit from a nice lady from the Social who told me she had scheduled some 'quiet time' for me in the local hospital, during which I was not to be disturbed and all my phone calls would be taken for me.

The nice lady from the Social asked me if there was anybody who should be notified of my temporary absence. A friend or family member, perhaps. No, I said, you see I am socially isolated. I have no close friends left who care about me and my one remaining family member is in an enclosed contemplative order of nuns in Southern Patagonia and, of course, I didn't want her disturbed on my account.

Liam O' Donnell

3

What Happens at a Psychiatric Consultation?

The general public's information about a psychiatric consultation is gleaned mostly from movies such as *Analyse This*, with a solemn-faced, bespectacled, bearded, psychiatrist listening to a gangster, sometimes lying on a couch, disclosing how he loved his mother. The psychiatrist doesn't ask questions, just makes the occasional observation, culminating in the gangster crying inconsolably and renouncing his evil ways, for the time being at least. To describe such a scenario as inaccurate is a grave understatement. The consultation is nothing like that: it is more structured and focused, with the specific goal of arriving at a working diagnosis and deciding on a treatment plan (Burns, 2014).

REFERRALS FOR ASSESSMENT BY A PSYCHIATRIST

You will require a referral from your GP to see a psychiatrist. Sometimes the referral may come from a hospital-based doctor, such as one based in the emergency department, if you have attended there, or from a surgeon or physician who may be involved in your treatment.

When the GP refers you as a public patient it will be to a psychiatrist who covers the geographic area in which you live. The reasons for this are administrative and are explained in Chapter 2. Alternatively, if you so wish, you can be referred to a private psychiatrist, without any geographic limitations.

You will see the doctor in the outpatient clinic in a hospital or health centre. Occasionally, if you are elderly or housebound, the consultation may take place in your own home.

EMERGENCY REFERRALS

Emergency referrals are made in acute and urgent circumstances, usually if there are concerns that the person is acutely psychotic or is a suicide or homicide risk. They will usually be made to the outpatient clinic. In the circumstances of such a referral, the initial contact may be with a psychiatric nurse and/or the junior doctor, who takes a history, followed by an interview with the consultant. From this a treatment plan will be provided.

The second route for urgent referrals is through the emergency departments. This route will be taken if there is no outpatient clinic that day, or if the referral is made outside normal working hours. This process differs slightly from the outpatient route. You will be seen on arrival by a nurse and triaged to a specialty (e.g. adult psychiatry) with an indicator of the urgency of the presentation. You will then be seen by the on-call psychiatric term doctor, or, if self-harm is the reason for referral, by a dedicated self-harm nurse specialist. This will be followed by a discussion with the responsible consultant psychiatrist and a decision regarding treatment and follow-up.

THE FIRST VISIT TO THE OUTPATIENT CLINIC

For a non-urgent referral, at the initial visit to a psychiatrist in the public health system, you will usually be seen initially by a psychiatrist-in-training. The initial interview may last an hour or sometimes longer: it depends on the complexity of your symptoms and problems. The history obtained will then be discussed with the consultant, whom you will then see unless they are absent for some reason (e.g. if they are attending to an emergency or on leave). Questions arising from the history will be clarified, and your diagnosis and possible treatments will be discussed. If the consultant is away, a consultant colleague should be covering their work and you may be seen by that person instead.

The myth that the patient is on a couch is commonplace, but this is not how any psychiatrist in Ireland treats their patients. When seen by a psychiatrist you will be sitting in a chair and the doctor may be at an angle to you or, less frequently, behind a desk directly opposite you.

If a close family member or friend has accompanied you, a separate interview with that person should be offered at the consultation. This interview is advisable, but it will not be done without your permission. Obtaining independent information is helpful in clarifying the impact that your symptoms have on your family, your work and your day-to-day living. A person who knows you well is in the best position to offer this information. The history you have given will not be shared with that individual, nor will the information they have given be shared with you. The interview with another person may also provide additional information about previous episodes of physical or psychiatric illness that you have forgotten about.

The combined history from you, from the GP, from your family member or friend, and from any previous medical records will help clarify:

1. if a psychiatric diagnosis is present;
2. what that diagnosis might be;
3. how severe is it in terms of its impact on your relationships and day-to-day functioning;
4. if you are at risk of harming yourself or anybody else;
5. what treatment is best for your constellation of symptoms and problems; and
6. if there are background factors that in themselves need attention from other mental health professionals, such as a psychologist or an occupational therapist.

WHAT QUESTIONS WILL I BE ASKED AT THE INITIAL INTERVIEW?

The initial interview with a person whom you most probably have never met is often very frightening. People sometimes tell me they didn't sleep for a few nights beforehand, they rehearsed what they would say (even though they have no idea what they will be asked), or they Googled the name of the consultant to reassure themselves that they are empathic, pleasant and thorough. These fears and uncertainties are perfectly understandable. For our part, we psychiatrists are cognisant of the reality that those whom we see are meeting a complete stranger and, over the course of an hour or so, that person is expected to open up their heart and mind to this stranger. This is a huge demand and expectation. The doctor's demeanour at the first interview may thus dictate how you will relate to your psychiatrist thereafter.

The interview will have two broad goals. The first is to get an overall understanding of your symptoms and your background so as to give a context to your problems. By that we mean why has this person developed these symptoms at this time? The second is to arrive at a diagnosis so that appropriate treatment can be offered.

The interview is wide ranging and may probe personal and intimate areas, depending on the reason for referral. If you referred with low mood, the questions will focus on symptoms and personal circumstances related to low mood. The psychiatrist is not there to judge but to offer an intervention to assist you.

All the information is confidential except in cases where there is a risk to you or to others. If sexual abuse is disclosed and the perpetrator is atill alive this must be reported to the relevant authorities. It is important to be forthcoming and honest: the more your psychiatrist knows, the better they will be able to understand your situation and respond with appropriate, evidence-based interventions.

AREAS OF INQUIRY

The areas about which questions will be asked are listed below.

Areas of Inquiry at Initial Assessment

- **History of presenting symptoms** – types, duration, frequency and severity. Specific symptoms will be asked about and their absence, as well as their presence, may be important: for example, sleep changes or weight loss.
- **Possible stressors or triggers** that the person thinks are relevant.
- **Family history** of physical and psychiatric illness. Family relationships.
- **Personal history** – early childhood, milestones, childhood trauma, schooling, employment, relationships (romantic or platonic).
- **Past and current physical and psychiatric conditions.** Medication and other treatments, past and present, for physical and psychiatric disorders.
- **Personality** before the onset of symptoms:

- Usual personality traits, e.g. dependent on others or confident, quick-tempered or placid
- Hobbies when well
- The presence or absence of social and other supports, such as religious beliefs and practices.
- Forensic history, i.e. offences, imprisonment or pending litigation

- **Mental state examination** – this is an examination of the doctor's own evaluation of symptoms rather than what the patient says. It will be considered under the following headings:
  - General appearance – tidy, dishevelled etc.
  - Speech – monotonous, monosyllabic, pressured, disorganised, etc.
  - Behaviour – slowed up, tremulous, obsessional etc.
  - Mood – anxious, sad, elated, normal (euthymic) etc.
  - Perception – hallucinations, illusions etc.
  - Thought content – delusions, obsessional ruminations, disorders of thought etc.
  - Control, suicidal ideation or plans etc.
  - Concentration – normal, inattentive etc.
  - Orientation – knows day, date, time, general news etc.
  - Insight – awareness of illness, of need for treatment, explanation for illness etc.

Reading through this list, you may think that more areas may be probed during the interview than you had expected. Psychiatrists are often asked, 'What have my education and my parents' relationship got to do with how I feel now?' And, indeed, the answer is often 'nothing', but sometimes these things can have a lot to do with how you feel. For instance, a person's family history of mental illness, or their having witnessed physical violence by a parent, may contribute to their current anger problems. Unless a wide number of areas is explored, it is likely that past events contributing to your current difficulties will be missed and treatment will then be less effective. *Psychopathology* is the term used to describe the emotions and mental processes that the person is experiencing.

The doctor may feel that certain aspects of your life are too sensitive to probe at a first interview and defer this until trust has been established. Indeed, nobody should be forced into opening up about something about which they are uncomfortable – although inevitably this may be necessary if the psychiatrist is to get a full picture and give you the best possible treatment. It is sometimes the case that failure to respond to treatment is due to a hidden issue lurking in the background. This may relate to alcohol misuse, childhood trauma or other 'personal secrets'. In asking about these the psychiatrist is not being inquisitive, but is trying to create a complete picture of you and your problems.

WHAT NEXT AFTER THE INITIAL ASSESSMENT?

At the end of the first evaluation in the outpatient clinic, the psychiatrist will usually recommend a course of treatment; it will be psychological, pharmacological or both. A psychological treatment such as cognitive therapy, and a pharmacological treatment such as an antidepressant, will be discussed. Of course, if no mental illness is present, you will be advised of this. The treatment recommendation will be followed by discussion with you and, if necessary, with the person accompanying you, and treatment will proceed only with your agreement. It may also be suggested that other mental health professionals are involved in your care, with home visits from the community mental health nurse, attendance at a day hospital for some hours on certain days, or referral to a psychologist for talking therapy or for further assessments, such as memory or personality assessments. If you have been having difficulties with work, an occupational therapist may be asked to establish the nature of the problems; if you are not working because of the severity of your illness, an evaluation of your ability to care for yourself, to budget and to do shopping may also be required. A social worker may be asked to assist with practical matters such as obtaining a medical card, a travel pass or other benefits. If your symptoms are interfering with work or education, you may be advised to take time off. Your GP will provide you with a certificate of sickness at the psychiatrist's request, and this should be given to your employer.

The psychiatrist, community mental health nurse, psychologist and occupational health therapist together comprise a team of mental health professionals known as the multidisciplinary team (MDT) – although not all teams are fortunate enough to have the full complement of members mentioned above. Others, that are well resourced, may additionally have music or art therapists, lifestyle coaches, family and relationship therapists and counsellors.

In the early stages of treatment your case will be discussed with the full team to consider which, if any, additional therapists or evaluations need to be involved in order to provide the widest possible response to your needs and treatment requirements.

On completion of the first interview you should be told what the likely diagnosis is, if possible. However, this may be unclear at this stage, and, if so, you should be advised of this. After the first interview a letter is usually sent to the referring doctor as to the working diagnosis and treatment plans.

Follow-up appointments will then be offered with one of the doctors (the junior doctor or consultant) and/or other members of the team, as required.

Occasionally, referral to the day hospital for more intensive evaluation and treatment is recommended. If you are acutely ill or actively suicidal, hospital admission would be recommended.

WHAT TREATMENTS MIGHT BE SUGGESTED?

The intervention you receive will depend on the diagnosis and on any background stressors contributing to your symptoms. You might be offered psychological or pharmacological interventions. The former is most commonly delivered by clinical psychologists or counsellors. Various psychotherapeutic approaches are available based on the different training processes and qualifications. Art therapy may sometimes be suggested. Psychoanalysis is seldom recommended nowadays. The most common therapies are CBT and DBT (see Chapter 1). Counselling, which refers to an approach of listening and support, may also be offered. (Counselling is the term used by the public for any form of talk therapy.)

Medication is used for some conditions, and for others a combination of psychological and pharmacological treatments is recommended. Prescriptions for medication may be written by the psychiatrist or junior doctor on the team, although for administrative reasons, some psychiatrists request that the GP actually writes the prescription, having advised them of the medication in writing after the consultation.

AREAS OF DISSATISFACTION AMONG PATIENTS

Patients frequently complain that at each appointment during the follow-up period they see a different doctor. This lack of continuity is a genuine and growing problem in Irish healthcare, and we must do better to give patients continuity of care. However, the health service faces many opposing demands, and increasing continuity is an uphill struggle. First, the consultant will not be in a position to see every patient due to the volume of work that would involve. After the initial consultation with a consultant, junior doctors take on the treatment of the patient, though they will remain in discussion with the consultant. Second, junior doctors are legally entitled to a 24-hour break after a night on call. This will inevitably impinge upon those attending a clinic. Third, junior doctors also take study leave and holiday breaks. Finally, the training in all specialties requires that each doctor moves to another consultant every six months in order to obtain experience in different sub-specialties or areas of interest.

A further concern for the patient that often arises during the consultation, particularly when permission is sought to interview a family member or somebody who knows the person well, is that personal information will be discussed. The patient may worry that issues regarding substance misuse, sexual orientation or behaviour will be discussed with this person. However, there is no ground for concern here: psychiatrists are legally and ethically bound to confidentiality. This is a serious responsibility, and confidentiality can be breached only in rare cases where there is a risk to the person's own safety and life or to that of others. This matter is discussed further in Chapter 12, under the heading Confidentiality.

WHAT ABOUT SEEING A PSYCHOLOGIST INSTEAD?

There is still something of a stigma attached to seeing a psychiatrist, and some ask why they could not have been referred to a psychologist instead. The distinction between psychiatry and psychology is a question that everybody raises. In general, psychology is the study and treatment of abnormal behaviour, although it may also study normal behaviour. Psychiatry, on the other hand, is defined as the study and treatment of mental illness. Psychology evolved from the arts and social sciences, while psychiatry evolved from medicine. This distinction is discussed further in Chapter 1.

PATIENT, CLIENT, SERVICE USER?

With an increasing focus on self-determination and autonomy in psychiatric practice and law, a question that has emerged in recent years is what those receiving healthcare should be called. The most enduring and common term is 'patient'. This has come under scrutiny, though, and some believe that it is paternalistic and implies passivity, and is thus disempowering. Suggested alternatives include 'client', 'consumer', 'customer', 'recipient' and 'service user'. However, these too have been criticised as implying a business-relationship model of healthcare that is too simple to capture the nature of the doctor-patient relationship. The debate has been particularly robust in psychiatry, though it has also touched other areas of medical practice.

In psychiatry, the upshot of this is that in administrative documents and even in common parlance among some mental health workers, the word 'patient' is avoided, and other terms, especially 'service user', are used. Nevertheless, most of those attending psychiatrists, or any other doctors, refer to themselves as patients. Perhaps this is simply custom and practice rather than preference. So what term do those we call 'patients' really prefer?

Many individual studies have examined this. The most comprehensive (Costa et al., 2019) is a 'meta-study' or systemic review of almost 46 peer-reviewed papers, and it found that among those with cancer, the term survivor was preferred, but that for most other patients (including mental health patients), 'patient' was the preferred term. So, for now, the term 'patient' is thriving.

BIBLIOGRAPHY

Burns, T. 'What to expect if you a re referred to a psychiatrist'. *Our Necessary Shadow: The Nature and Meaning of Psychiatry*. London: Penguin. 2014.

Costa, S., DSJ, Mercieca-Bebber, R., Tesson, S., Seidler, Z. et al. 'Patient, client, consumer, survivor or other alternatives? A scoping review of preferred terms for labelling individuals who access healthcare across settings'. *BMJ Open*. 9; e025166. 2019.

A success story – from patient to therapist

I am passionate about recovery and believe that as we learn about ourselves and develop healthy relationships we can lead a happy and contented life and in a way cure ourselves of our mental illness. I may sound arrogant but I would be prepared to be assessed by a psychiatrist today and my guess is they would not diagnose any mental illness.

I am 66 years of age now. In 1974 I was hospitalised with a psychotic episode and diagnosed with schizophrenia. In 1976, on my second admission, I was diagnosed with schizoaffective disorder. On my third admission, in 1980, I was diagnosed with bipolar disorder. I was also admitted in 1984, 1986, 1988 and 1990. Prior to each admission I stopped taking my medication, precipitating a further psychotic episode. In 2008 I finally succeeded. I came off all psychiatric medication and have good mental health without any further admissions since.

I have been on a voyage of discovery since I had my first episode as an immature and very self-conscious 19-year-old. I am no longer afraid of madness. I have learnt a lot about myself by reflecting on my delusional thinking and my hallucinations. They seem similar to dreams and can always be connected to issues that I have struggled with in my life. Probably more like nightmares than dreams that I did not wake up from but struggled with until I ended up in hospital again.

Following my first admission I was training as a Samaritan volunteer and a local psychiatrist gave us a lecture on mental Illness. He described schizophrenia as a 'disintegrating personality' and suggested that it would not be very worth while to listen to such people if they called our Samaritan branch as they were no-hopers (my words). Not very encouraging when I was trying to make a life for myself following my diagnosis. I remained a Samaritan volunteer for the next six years, moving to the Dublin branch when I secured a place in social work training at Trinity College in 1980. Prior to securing this place I applied for psychiatric nursing in two Irish hospitals and one English hospital. I did not secure a place in the Irish hospitals. When interviewed for the English hospital I was told I was successful, but when I filled in a questionnaire on my medical history they wrote back saying a place was no longer available to me.

I learned to keep my mental illness a secret, believing that I needed to do so in order to succeed in life. Just prior to my graduation in social work in 1984 I had my fourth episode. Despite getting an honours degree I was unsure about getting my professional qualification. My college tutor advocated on my behalf and I was allowed to graduate with a professional social work qualification.

I worked for what is now X for three years, Y for eighteen months, Z for three years. I resigned from each job following my fifth, sixth and seventh psychotic episodes, as I felt I was now tarnished and that I would not succeed in that occupation. In 1987 I applied to train as a psychotherapist, giving my own mental illness as my motivation for the course, but did not secure a place. In 1990 I joined the probation service and completed a master's in equality studies (1992–94). I worked in probation for the following 18 years, completing a further master's In family psychotherapy (2000–3). When applying for this second master's I did not disclose my history of mental illness and secured one of the 12 places available out of over 60 people attending for interview. In 2009 I took early retirement from A service (the government early retirement scheme). In 2011 I secured work with a local charity called the BRF Project, and continue to work there. I pride myself on having a very good sick leave record despite my hospitalisations for mental illness.

I don't want my story to sound bitter because I experienced some discrimination over the years. I got married in 1995 and remain happily married. I enjoy life and consider myself quite fit, running three times a week. I cycle to work and am a member of a community choir. I am involved in some voluntary mental health activity. One of my sources of healing over the years has been voluntary work, mostly in the area of mental health. My strategy was to keep my mental illness a secret for fear of discrimination up to my retirement from the probation service. I now talk openly about my mental illness and my recovery to anyone who will listen. In 2015 I published my memoir, *Embracing Sanity*. (The 400 copies are all sold out but some copies still are available in libraries.)

4

Stress- and Stressor-related Disorders

WHAT IS STRESS?

Stress is a confusing term because it is used in different ways in day-to-day parlance.

The medical definition of stress is that it is the reaction of people to situations or events that threaten to disrupt or harm their physical or psychological well-being. Some definitions include their psychosocial or psychospiritual well-being also. The word 'stressor' refers to the triggering event or situation: a stressor is that which causes stress.

The diagram below is a simple illustration of the most stressful events identified in the scientific literature.

Stressor and response

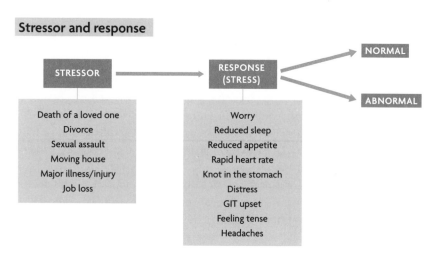

It can be seen that the types of stressor are many, and the list above is not exhaustive. It also shows that the response to a stressor may be normal or abnormal.

Some of the stress symptoms listed above may be present even in normal adaptive stress responses. These are considered abnormal if their impact is excessive and causes a fall-off in day-to-day functioning.

There is a tendency to assume that the stress response is always negative, but in fact responding to stressful events by becoming stressed may be normal and even beneficial. An example of this is given here.

Case Vignette

John is preparing for his final examination for his arts degree. He is worrying a lot about the examination and has lost his appetite. His weight has dropped perhaps by 1 kg. He sometimes lies awake planning what he needs to revise the following day but mostly his sleep is fine. As the examination approaches, he begins to put in more work, up to five hours study per day. He usually takes Saturday off and may meet friends in the evening. His parents are worried that he is overdoing things, as he seems to be preoccupied about doing well. He tells them that he is fine and that he is able to retain what he is studying.

Comment:
The stressor is the anticipation of the examination. As John gets more 'psyched up' about the exam he begins to work harder. His family fear that he is overdoing things and should ease off a little.

Clearly the number of hours of study is only part of the answer to whether John is working to excess or not. The best way to establish if his stress response is helpful or harmful is to check if he is functioning normally. Is his concentration OK? Is he retaining what he reads? Is he sleeping well generally? Is he able to get up in the mornings and go to the library to study or to his revision lectures? Is he experiencing panic or feeling overwhelmed?

In John's case there do not appear to be any abnormalities in his day-to-day functioning. Had he studied for less time every day, arguably he might not have done as well as he was hoping to. He was driving himself hard, to be sure, but showed no signs of being abnormally stressed, and the stressor acted as a stimulus to allow him to work to his capacity.

Of importance in John's case is that this is a time-limited response because it has occurred in the context of exams. If it had occurred as a result of unemployment and been prolonged it might ultimately have led to difficulties in day-to-day functioning and become abnormal.

Note: This is not a real case, but it describes a typical scenario.

Whatever the stressor, if our ability to look after those who need us, such as our children or other family members, is impaired, or our ability to meet others as we did previously lessens, or our efficiency at work is reduced as a consequence of the symptoms caused by the stressor, then our response is likely to be in the abnormal range. It is our day-to-day functioning that tells us whether we are experiencing normal or abnormal stress.

It is tempting to assume that anybody exposed to a major stressor might react in a negative way, but most people come through the most difficult of stressful events with little or no need for any professional help in dealing with their distress. Provided we have people to talk to about the stressor who can advise us on how to deal with our situation, no further help is required when we are faced with the stressors of everyday life. Of course, if we have nobody to support us, we may need to see a therapist to help us through, even though our reaction is not abnormal.

Sometimes short-term medication can help with sleep loss, but generally no intervention is necessary. Increasingly there is concern that the problems of everyday life are being medicalised, and that both medication and talking therapies are supplanting the resources we have within ourselves and the help we can receive from our friends and families (Horowitz and Wakefield, 2007). Professional help is usually only needed when a stress response is abnormal.

HOW CAN I TELL IF MY RESPONSE TO A STRESSFUL EVENT IS ABNORMAL?

When people are responding excessively to stress, their day-to-day functioning deteriorates. So the person may withdraw from social situations, in the workplace they will notice that they are less productive, those in education will miss assignments and even not attend class, and homemakers will find themselves less able to tend to their children, do the cooking and so on. In the business world, if people have to work under excessive strain, for example when the relationship between worker and management is disturbed, stress levels become so high that performance falls off and absenteeism results. This then compounds the original stress response.

Symptoms such as anxiety, poor appetite and reduced concentration due to worry may also occur, but these can be part of a normal response, so change in day-to-day functioning is the clearest indicator that the response is excessive.

The relationship between response to a stressor and behaviour is illustrated below. This graph is called the Yerkes-Dodson curve after the two psychologists, Robert M. Yerks and H. M. Dodson, who described this relationship in 1908.

Yerkes-Dodson Law

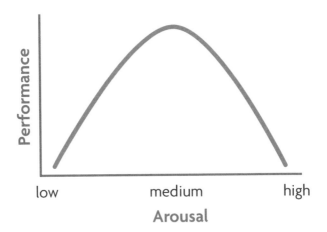

This figure graphs the relationship between the stressfulness of a situation (on the horizontal axis) and a person's performance while subject to this level of stress (on the vertical axis). The graph shows that as mental and physiological arousal (anxiety) increase in response to the stressor, performance/functioning improves until it reaches a tipping point (the top of the curve). As stressor intensity continues to increase after this point, performance (functioning) decreases. In simple language, this shows that everybody has a breaking point, which varies from person to person. Some people can withstand a lot of pressure, while for others symptoms of abnormal stress and malfunction occur with low levels of pressure.

Since stressful events and a stress response are part and parcel of humankind, the implication of the Yerkes-Dodson curve is that attempting to rid our world of stress would lead to humanity falling short of its goals; this is because the arousal that is needed to spur us to action would not exist. On the other hand, if the stress level became too high people would become incapacitated and performance would also fall off. We flourish best while slightly stressed, and so although we need not aspire to be constantly slightly stressed, we should not try to eradicate stress from human life altogether.

WHAT FACTORS INFLUENCE HOW I RESPOND TO STRESSORS?

The factors that influence this are listed below. These are called moderators.

Influences on response to stressors

Poor response/vulnerability	Positive response/resilience
• Childhood abuse, neglect, bullying	• Loving/protective familial environment
• Parental loss	• Parental stability
• Poor familial and social supports	• Strong familial and social supports
• Absence of confidants	• Presence of one or more confidants
• Absence of a religious or other structured belief system	• Presence of religious beliefs or structured spiritual practices

- Coping using avoidance – 'It'll go away'
- Low self-confidence
- Being an innate worrier and highly strung
- Using alcohol and other substances to cope
- Using social supports for catharsis, i.e. emotion-focused coping
- Prior difficulties with stress, e.g. required professional help, self-harm behaviours

- Coping using approach (facing up)
- High self-confidence
- Being innately calm even under pressure
- Using exercise, some distraction, e.g. reading, to cope
- Using social supports for problem solving, i.e. instrumental coping
- Prior coping with stress, i.e. not requiring professional help

Personality is one of the key influences on how people react to stressful events. So those who are by nature calm, who have high self-esteem and who face problems and seek practical solutions are more likely to respond in an adaptive, positive manner than those who have low self-regard or who have experienced childhood trauma, and who avoid the problem by refusing to consider it, perhaps even abusing alcohol or drugs to help the avoidant defence. As well as a person's own personality, another important factor in stress response is having people to discuss the problem with in order to obtain advice. Having interests and hobbies that will distract you from ongoing worry and refocus you on other things is a helpful moderator, as is having religious beliefs and engaging in religious or spiritual practices such as prayer and meditation (Lorenz et al., 2019). Exercise is also of benefit since it releases the individual's own store of opiates, known as endorphins, and it also helps reduce inflammation and promotes growth of the brain cells.

You also need to consider how you coped in the past with stressors. Most people will be exposed to many stressful events in the course of their life, and if you generally manage the stress response and cope well with it, the likelihood is that the same will happen this time. The ability to draw on the resources available to you, either 'internal' (your personality and religious/spiritual beliefs), or 'external' (e.g. friends, family and community), is known as *resilience*. This has recently received a lot of attention in the scientific community of psychiatrists and psychologists.

Stressors may be acute or chronic. *Acute* stressors can arise at any time and without warning; for example, unexpected loss of a loved one or the sudden loss of one's job. *Chronic* stressors include long-term unemployment, financial problems or relationship or health difficulties. These types of stressors are all common in our world, and it is the make-up of the individual and their social supports that determines whether a person faced with these stressors will react to them in a proportionate or disproportionate manner. The one thing all stress responses have in common will be the presence of symptoms, but whether day-to-day functioning will be changed is what will separate healthy from unhealthy responses.

DO ABNORMAL STRESS REACTIONS HAVE A NAME?

There are several recognised psychiatric conditions that are caused by stressors.

The first of these conditions is called adjustment disorder (AjD), which refers to exaggerated stress responses that are triggered by an event. The term 'trigger' is key: it means that the symptoms and their associated negative impact on day-to-day activities would not have occurred without the triggering event. In adjustment disorder, in many respects these reactions are understandable, but they are *excessive* in the impact they have on the individual's functioning.

The symptoms are similar to those in normal stress, but they are more intense: low mood, worry about one's predicament, sadness, anxiety, concentration difficulties, irritability, insomnia, reduced appetite and anger are prominent and present in various combinations. At times the person may have suicidal thoughts or may feel hopeless, and they may act on these by self-harming. AjD is particularly common in people who have serious physical illnesses such as cancer, or those who sustain serious physical injuries. Bullying in the workplace is another common trigger. Depending on the dominant symptoms, the disorder is classified into several subtypes:

- AjD with depressed mood
- AjD with anxiety
- AjD with mixed anxiety and depression
- AjD with disturbance of conduct

- AjD with mixed disturbance of emotions and conduct
- Unspecified AjD

The depressed subtype may be misdiagnosed as a depressive illness (termed depressive episode or major depression), which is discussed in Chapter 6, or as an anxiety disorder, which is discussed in Chapter 5. The basic difference between AjD and these two conditions is that, unlike depressive illness or generalised anxiety, AjD is triggered by some specific stressor, whereas the others can occur with or without any trigger (see Chapters 5 and 7).

Let us look at the time-line and symptoms of an episode of AjD. The symptoms begin following a stressful event. They may not appear immediately, but they will normally appear within a few days or weeks. They fluctuate depending on whether the person is exposed to reminders of the stressor, e.g. by talking about it or attending meetings in relation to it, and this results in distress. Mood and related symptoms revert to normal when the person is removed from the stressor. When dealing with the stressor directly, the person may feel not just anxious, but overwhelmed and unable to cope. They may require time off work or college, and if they are a carer for their family may need help with that. The symptoms last as long as the stressor or its consequences. Symptoms resolve once either of these ends, or if the person is removed from the environment triggering the reaction. For example, a person who is being bullied at work and is diagnosed with an AjD will improve when they have time off work on holiday or sick leave, but the symptoms will recur when they return to that work environment if no changes have been made there to alleviate the bullying.

WHAT HELP IS AVAILABLE FOR AJD?

The main approach to treatment is using one of the talking therapies to help the person adapt to the stressor. This may be cognitive or problem-solving therapy. Where possible, the person should be encouraged to make changes in their life so as to distance themselves from the trigger. In some circumstances, though, this may unfortunately not be possible. For example, a person being bullied at work may not be able to leave that job because they may not be able to find a new job if they do leave. A more practical approach here would include, for instance, approaching HR to bring the difficulties to the attention of management. The symptoms of anxiety, low mood and perhaps anger that may be present can be helped by mindfulness, relaxation exercises and general exercise.

Because of the frequency of mood changes, this group is often mistakenly thought to have depressive illness or generalised anxiety, and they may be prescribed antidepressants. However, there is no evidence that these improve low mood in those with this condition. Short-term medication such as sleeping tablets and/or antianxiety medication may be helpful, as this may help insomnia and anxiety symptoms; however, to properly treat this condition, psychological treatment is recommended. If the symptoms continue even after the stressor and its consequences have been removed, then the person may have tipped into depressive illness (see Chapter 6), but in most people the symptoms resolve and the person is able to get on with life again.

Case Vignette

Mr X, a 35-year-old man, was seen by a passer-by standing on a bridge at 6.30 in the evening. The passer-by asked Mr X why he was there and he said he was about to jump in the river because he had lost his job a few weeks earlier and that his wife and children were suffering as a result. Money was very short and he had failed to secure a new job. The passer-by talked him down and persuaded him to come to the emergency department, where he was evaluated psychiatrically and admitted to the psychiatric unit in the hospital.

He said that he had left a suicide note in his car. He reported increasingly low mood and hopelessness since the loss of his job. Debt was mounting and he and his family were dependent on charities for assistance. He feared he would lose his home due to problems meeting the mortgage, with which his parents and siblings were helping. Seeing no solution to his debts he decided to end his life. He had weeks of sleeplessness and impaired concentration. He had 8 kg weight loss due to worry, and had lost interest in looking for work. His concentration was poor due to his constant worry about his predicament. He had no history of any prior mental or physical health problems.

During his stay in hospital he was not given any medication apart from sleeping tablets for the first two nights. He was reported to be eating well, attending all activities and engaging in conversation with staff and fellow patients. His mood was not noted to be depressed although he was extremely worried about his predicament. He reported relief that his life had been saved and enjoyed seeing his family during visiting time.

The social worker referred him to a free financial advice service for help in addressing his debts, and he was also helped in signing up for the state assistance schemes to which he was entitled. He was linked in with retraining programmes. The psychologist offered him therapy using problem-solving techniques. He began to discuss his problems more openly with the therapists and was discharged two weeks post-admission. Throughout the period of follow-up he remained symptom free and continued the process of resolving his debt and employment problems. He was discharged to his GP six months post-admission and did not require medication at any point after discharge.

Comment:

This gentleman's history showed that the onset of symptoms was closely related to being made redundant. His increasing hopelessness and sense of helplessness led to him to being on the point of a serious suicide attempt. Once he was in an environment that removed him from his adverse circumstances and which offered practical assistance and emotional support, his symptoms resolved rapidly with psychological therapy. This case study indicates that AjD can persist while adverse social circumstances continue and also that it can, in some instances, be associated with near-miss suicide. This history illustrates the superficial overlap between AjD and depression: this gentleman might easily have been prescribed antidepressants as he had symptoms almost identical to those with depressive illness, when in fact his symptoms were driven exclusively by his circumstances and resolved when he was offered practical and emotional support.

Note: This is not a real case but based on the features of many cases that the author has treated.

Post-traumatic stress disorder (PTSD) is another condition that is triggered by stressful events. It has a different group of symptoms from AjD and the trigger is more serious.

This was previously called 'shellshock' and was particularly common during the First World War when soldiers returned from the trenches so traumatised by the fighting and shelling that they seemed to be in constant disengagement from life. The novel *Regeneration* (1991), by Pat Barker, is set during the First World War in an Edinburgh psychiatric hospital specialising in treating this condition. Barker recreated the characters of the war poets Wilfred Owen and Siegfried Sassoon in this acclaimed work. In some cultures, even those that are war-torn, the frequency with which PTSD is diagnosed is low, and it is thought that this is because the symptoms are accepted by stalwart citizens as an inevitable consequence of conflict rather than indicating a psychiatric disorder requiring treatment.

The term 'PTSD' was coined after the Vietnam War, when large numbers of veterans had the symptoms that define the condition. Giving it a name that encapsulated trauma as causing a disorder was seen by some as an attempt at appeasing anti-Vietnam War campaigners. Thereafter, the conditions in which it was diagnosed expanded to include bullying in the workplace or even being given bad news in an unsympathetic manner. At a certain point it became clear that the condition was being diagnosed far too liberally, and the criteria for symptoms required to diagnose PTSD have since become much more tightly defined.

In legal circles the term 'nervous shock' is still used to refer to PTSD, but this is a legal and not a psychiatric term. It implies that the manner in which the trauma occurred is the cause of the symptoms, by generating a shock to the psyche. This concept is not accepted within psychiatry.

STRESSFUL VS TRAUMATIC EVENTS

The events that trigger PTSD are of much greater severity than those triggering AjD. Here the distinction between *stressful* and *traumatic* events is important. *Stressful* events are those of lesser severity and are common in day-to-day life. They include such things as relationship problems, divorce, and job loss. Most people do not respond to them pathologically such that their day-to-day functioning is impaired, and while they cause unhappiness and worry, psychiatric disorder is not inevitable. If people in these situations do develop a psychiatric disorder it may be AjD, described above, or a depressive illness (see Chapter 7).

Traumatic events, on the other hand, are such that most people would be very upset by them and, even in the most resilient people, these events may cause reactions with great mental suffering, although those who are by nature anxious or worriers are at higher risk.

The crucial consideration is the *severity* of the traumatic event. These must be 'exceptionally threatening or catastrophic' (WHO, 1994), and typical examples include being exposed to death, being threatened with death, receiving an actual or threatened serious injury, or being a victim of actual or threatened sexual violence. The WHO definition includes direct exposure, as well as learning that a relative or close friend was exposed to or witnessed such an event. Viewing the images, captured on television and reproduced in newspapers, of the 1989 Hillsborough disaster in Liverpool, when 89 people were trampled to death in a football stadium, is a typical example of witnessing a traumatic event.

In the past, the major consideration determining whether PTSD was diagnosed was the person's own evaluation of the impact of the trauma on them. This personalised approach meant that if a relatively minor event, such as a car accident with no physical injury and little visible damage to the vehicle, was claimed to be perceived by the person as having put their life at risk, this claim would be accepted at face value. This has now changed, and the events must now actually be threatening to health or life for a diagnosis of PTSD to be made. This change has come about in response to the over-diagnosis of the condition, particularly in the context of likely false attestations of trauma in legal litigation following accidents.

Four main symptom clusters are present in PTSD and these are summarised in the table below. More detail is provided in the Appendix to this chapter.

> ### Symptom clusters in PTSD
>
> PTSD symptoms are clustered into the following four groups:
> 1. The person relives the event if reminded of it.
> 2. The person avoids reminders of the event.
> 3. The person has excessive anxiety regarding the event and is over-alert to danger, is irritabile and/or is easily startled.
> 4. The person has negative thoughts about the event (such as excessively blaming themselves for it) , or have difficulty recalling it.

Note: The above refers to the American (DSM) system of diagnosis. The WHO system used in Europe has three clusters. See the Appendix to this chapter for specific details of symptoms in the DSM and WHO criteria.

As a consequence of the distressing and incapacitating symptoms of PTSD, people may drink alcohol to excess, develop depressive symptoms, and harm themselves by cutting or overdosing. Relationships with loved ones often become strained due to the person's detachment, and social withdrawal from family and other events may occur.

Trauma that is persistent and particularly horrifying, such as childhood abuse, genocide or torture, can lead to a more difficult to treat type of trauma, now referred to as *complex PTSD* (see the Appendix to this chapter).

Most people exposed to traumatic events do not develop PTSD. Some are able to get on with their lives without any significant lasting effects of the trauma, while others develop other conditions, such as AjD (discussed above) or a depressive episode (see page 99).

HOW COMMON IS PTSD AND WHEN DOES IT OCCUR?

PTSD is more common after manmade than natural disasters. It is possible that this is because it destroys our trust in human beings like ourselves. How could we do this to one another? However, this explanation remains a hypothesis for the moment. It also occurs frequently in first responders to a major event, such as fire or police officers, and in paramedics attending fatal road accidents or serious assaults.

What happens to the brain with PTSD?

Biological changes have been identified in association with PTSD, along with abnormalities in certain areas of the brain. These are called the amygdala and hippocampus and the lateral septum in the prefrontal cortex. They have been described using imaging studies.

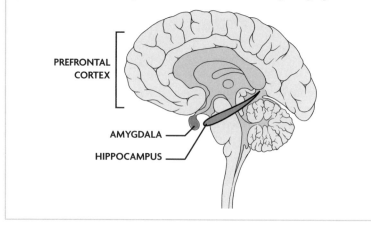

PREFRONTAL CORTEX

AMYGDALA —

HIPPOCAMPUS —

The lifetime prevalence (frequency) of PTSD in the US population is estimated to be 3.6% among men and 9.7% among women (Kessler, 2005). Measures over the previous month find figures of 1.8% among men and 5.2% among women. In general the figures are very difficult to interpret since they vary depending on when the study was carried out, on which continent, in which population (the general population, war zone veterans or victims of violence or traffic accidents), and whether data was based on lifetime rates or one-month rates.

It is worth remembering that until 2013 the threshold for making the diagnosis was quite low. It was the person themselves who decided what was a traumatic event and what was not. This was tightened in DSM-5 (American Psychiatric Association, 2013) which specified the types of event that could be regarded as traumatic. This change will also make a difference to the prevalence in the direction of reduction.

In the early period after a traumatic event it is common for people to experience symptoms similar to those of PTSD. For example, following the 9/11 attack on the World Trade Center in New York, symptoms matching those of PTSD were present in over 7% of the population five to seven weeks after the event, but dropped to 0.6% nine months later. A diagnosis of PTSD is not made for at least four weeks after the event because it is recognised that there are short-term responses to traumas that improve quickly, as happened post 9/11. These early symptoms are known as acute stress disorder (ASD). In the majority of people these symptoms improve within weeks.

WHAT TREATMENTS CAN I GET?

Treatment of PTSD is normally done through a combination of medication and psychological treatment. The family of antidepressants known as SSRIs are the most common to be used for the treatment of PTSD. These include sertraline, escitalopram and venlafaxine.

Psychological therapies such as trauma-focused therapy, a type of cognitive therapy, are also common. Eye movement desensitisation and reprocessing (EMDR), first described in 1989, is one of the newer and lesser-known treatments. Although we do not know how it works, it appears to help patients with the processing of flashbacks and traumatic memories. It is one of the main treatments recommended in 2018 by the UK-based National Institute of Clinical Excellence (NICE) for non-combat related trauma.

Many people ask about Critical Incident Stress Debriefing (CISD). This is a type of group therapy in which the individuals describe the event and their emotions in order to try to process them. This was sometimes used after traumatic events in the workplace such as were experienced by soldiers in war zones and health personnel witnessing traumatic deaths. The rationale was that it may help prevent PTSD by helping the person process and achieve perspective on the event in a supportive environment with others similarly exposed. However, it has been found to be more harmful than beneficial and it is no longer recommended by NICE (2018).

WHAT ABOUT GRIEF?

Grief is a normal response to the loss of a loved one. It may be more severe if the person dies unexpectedly, traumatically, or is a child. It is characterised by deep sadness, tearfulness, yearning, sometimes guilt, and at times yearning for the loved one. Sometimes the loved one is momentarily 'seen' in the faces of others. Occasionally the bereaved person may even deny that their loved one has gone and sets a place at the table for them. Most people gradually adapt to life without their loved one, although this can be frightening too as the person fears they will forget them. This, of course, will not happen, since loved ones are never forgotten, but the bereaved do adapt to the loss.

Some people do not grieve, or at least won't allow themselves grieve, usually through fear of losing control. Looking at pictures of the loved one, visiting the grave, 'talking' to the person or watching videos of them can unleash the pent-up emotions. If the person is unwilling to engage in these activities and uses avoidance techniques, then the normal grief process remains inhibited and unresolved. This inhibited grief can result in depressive illness or unexplained physical symptoms.

The acute phase of grief lasts about six months, although there is much variation between individuals. It may continue with less intensity for a few years, and many still cry about the loss even years later, for instance on special occasions such as family weddings, anniversaries etc. Grief is more difficult if for some reason the person cannot process their emotions. For example, if a victim of a road traffic accident, in which a loved one lost their life, is trying to cope with their own major surgery from injuries received in the crash, they may be unable to focus on the loss of their loved one. If the relationship with the deceased was secret or improper in some way, the griever's emotions may also be curtailed.

For years the theory dominating grief was set out by Elisabeth Kübler-Ross in *Death and Dying*, in which she identified 'the five stages of grief.' These stages are denial, anger, bargaining, depression and acceptance. Kübler-Ross's theory was hugely influential, but it was also too prescriptive. Many people believed they were not grieving properly if they did not experience the phases set out by her. Newer approaches recognise that grief may not occur in accordance with these stages. A more recent theory, known as 'continuing bonds' (Klasman, 2018), is probably a better model of grief. This theory states that people continue to have a bond with the deceased by talking to them, keeping mementos, carrying pictures and so on. In general, interrupting the natural grieving process can be damaging to a person and prevent their healing, and this is one of the reasons why bereavement counselling for those experiencing normal grief is not recommended.

Grief is abnormal when the acute features persist beyond the usual six-month period *and* when the person is not functioning after the feelings of sadness would be expected to have lessened, which is after a few years. Refusing to mention the deceased may also be indicative of an abnormal reaction. The circumstances of the loss also play a role in the depth and duration of the grief: Was the death particularly horrific? Was the deceased a child? How has the bereaved coped with death in the past? Additionally, the expression of grief varies across cultures, and in some cultures grief may be more publicly exhibited than in others. These factors need to be taken into account when evaluating whether a particular individual is showing a normal or pathological response to the loss. If, in light of all the above, you think your or someone else's grief is pathological, then you might consider counselling, which is beneficial in dealing with abnormal grief.

If symptoms associated with depressive illness, such as low mood, insomnia, impaired concentration and panic attacks persist, and if day-to-day functioning is impaired, the person may have developed a depressive episode (major depression) and also require antidepressants. There is concern that normal grief has been medicalised and wrongly transformed into a psychiatric disorder (Horowitz and Wakefield, 2007).

Features of grief that are mistakenly thought of as being pathological

- Not experiencing the five phases (see above)
- Talking to the deceased
- Hearing the deceased speaking
- Seeing the deceased in other people in crowds
- Becoming upset years after the loss, on specific occasions
- Wearing an item of clothing belonging to the deceased

Among the factors that protect against abnormal grief reactions are having religious beliefs, engaging fully in the funeral and having friends, confidants and social supports to turn to. As such, close family members should attend the funeral of their loved one unless there are grave reasons not to. Speaking about the deceased also helps since it facilitates the expression of sadness.

IS DEPRESSIVE ILLNESS A STRESSOR-RELATED DISORDER?

Depressive illness is not included in the stressor-related group of disorders described above since it can also occur with any stressor. It is recognised that depressive illness can be triggered by life events such as loss of a loved one through death, as described above. Other possible triggers include redundancy, loss of pets, marital breakdown or childbirth, to mention just a few. However, it can also occur without any stressor, and arguably does so in the majority of cases. The key symptoms in this group are early morning wakening and worsening mood in the morning (see Chapter 7). Since a stressor is not an essential requirement for triggering a depressive illness, this is *not* regarded as a stressor-related condition. Those conditions described in this chapter, namely AjD, PTSD, and abnormal grief, all *do* require a specific event to have occurred shortly before the onset of symptoms. Without the stressor these diagnoses cannot be made.

 WHAT YOU CAN DO FOR YOURSELF AND WHAT OTHERS CAN DO FOR YOU

- Share your worries about the event with a confidant.
- Seek practical guidance and advice on how to deal with your predicament.
- Be proactive rather than passive in dealing with your situation
- Talk to others who may have been in a similar situation.
- Avoid using alcohol or illegal drugs to help you cope.
- When you are bereaved speak about your loved one – do not avoid reminders of the deceased.

APPENDIX 1

Criteria for PTSD in DSM-5 (APA) and ICD-11 (WHO)

———

DSM-5 CRITERIA FOR PTSD

Criterion A (one required): The person was exposed to: death, threatened death, actual or threatened serious injury, or actual or threatened sexual violence, in the following way(s):

- Direct exposure
- Witnessing the trauma
- Learning that a relative or close friend was exposed to a trauma
- Indirect exposure to aversive details of the trauma, usually in the course of professional duties (e.g. first responders, medics)

Criterion B (one required): The traumatic event is persistently re-experienced, in the following way(s):

- Unwanted upsetting memories
- Nightmares
- Flashbacks
- Emotional distress after exposure to traumatic reminders
- Physical reactivity after exposure to traumatic reminders

Criterion C (one required): Avoidance of trauma-related stimuli after the trauma, in the following way(s):

- Trauma-related thoughts or feelings
- Trauma-related reminders

Criterion D (two required): Negative thoughts or feelings that began or worsened after the trauma, in the following way(s):

- Inability to recall key features of the trauma

- Overly negative thoughts and assumptions about oneself or the world
- Exaggerated blame of self or others for causing the trauma
- Negative affect
- Decreased interest in activities
- Feeling isolated
- Difficulty experiencing positive affect

Criterion E (two required): Trauma-related arousal and reactivity that began or worsened after the trauma, in the following way(s):
- Irritability or aggression
- Risky or destructive behaviour
- Hypervigilance
- Heightened startle reaction
- Difficulty concentrating
- Difficulty sleeping

Criterion F (required): Symptoms last for more than one month.

Criterion G (required): Symptoms create distress or functional impairment (e.g. social, occupational).

Criterion H (required): Symptoms are not due to medication, substance use, or other illness.

Two specifications:
- **Dissociative specification.** In addition to meeting criteria for diagnosis, an individual experiences high levels of either of the following in reaction to trauma-related stimuli:
    - **Depersonalisation.** Experience of being an outside observer or detached from oneself (e.g. feeling as if 'this is not happening to me', or as if one were in a dream).
    - **Derealisation.** Experience of unreality, distance or distortion (e.g. 'things are not real').
- **Delayed specification.** Full diagnostic criteria are not met until at least six months after the trauma(s), although onset of symptoms may occur immediately.

ICD-11 PTSD

PTSD may develop following exposure to an extremely threatening or horrific event or series of events. It is characterised by all of the following: (1) re-experiencing the traumatic event or events in the present in the form of vivid intrusive memories, flashbacks or nightmares. Re-experiencing may occur via one or multiple sensory modalities and is typically accompanied by strong or overwhelming emotions, particularly fear or horror, and strong physical sensations; (2) avoidance of thoughts and memories of the event or events, or avoidance of activities, situations or people reminiscent of the event(s); and (3) persistent perceptions of heightened current threat, for example as indicated by hypervigilance or an enhanced startle reaction to stimuli such as unexpected noises. The symptoms persist for at least several weeks and cause significant impairment in personal, family, social, educational, occupational or other important areas of functioning.

ICD-11 COMPLEX PTSD

Complex post-traumatic stress disorder (Complex PTSD) is a disorder that may develop following exposure to an event or series of events of an extremely threatening or horrific nature, most commonly prolonged or repetitive events from which escape is difficult or impossible (e.g. torture, slavery, genocide campaigns, prolonged domestic violence, repeated childhood sexual or physical abuse). All diagnostic requirements for PTSD are met. In addition, Complex PTSD is characterised by severe and persistent (1) problems in affect regulation; (2) beliefs about oneself as diminished, defeated or worthless, accompanied by feelings of shame, guilt or failure related to the traumatic event; and (3) difficulties in sustaining relationships and in feeling close to others. These symptoms cause significant impairment in personal, family, social, educational, occupational or other important areas of functioning.

BIBLIOGRAPHY

Diagnostic and statistical manual of mental disorders, 5th ed. Washington, DC: American Psychiatric Association. 2013.

Casey, P. *Adjustment Disorder: From Controversy to Clinical Practice*. Oxford: Oxford University Press. 2018.

Barker, P. *Regeneration*. London: Penguin. 1991.

Horowitz, A. V. and Wakefield, J. C. *The Loss of Sadness: How Psychiatry Transformed Normal Sorrow into Depressive Disorder*. New York, NY: Oxford University Press. 2007.

Kessler, R. C., Berglund, P., Delmer, O. et al. 'Lifetime prevalence and age-of-onset distributions of *DSM-IV* disorders in the National Comorbidity Survey Replication'. *Archives of General Psychiatry,* 62(6): 593–602. 2005.

Klass, D., Silverman, P., Nickman, S. et al. *Continuing Bonds: New Understandings of Grief*. Abingdon: Taylor & Francis. 1996.

Lorenz, L., Doherty, A., and Casey, P., 'The Role of Religion in Buffering the Impact of Stressful Life Events on Depressive Symptoms in Patients with Depressive Episodes or Adjustment Disorder'. *International Journal of Environmental Research and Public Health*. 16 July 2019.

National Institute for Health and Care Excellence (NICE). 'Post-traumatic stress disorder' (NICE Quality Standard No. 116). 2018.

World Health Organisation. *International Classification of Diseases*, 11th ed. Geneva: WHO. 2019.

USEFUL RESOURCES

From stress to resilience | Raphael Rose | TEDxManhattanBeach YouTube

Barry, Harry. *Toxic Stress: A step-by-step guide to managing stress*. London: Orion Spring. 2017.

5

Anxiety and Fear-related Disorders

As described in Chapter 4, anxiety can, sometimes and in moderation, be a helpful if not pleasant emotion. Symptoms of anxiety are known to everybody: we all feel anxious at certain times in our lives. For example, before performing on stage many actors and musicians will experience performance anxiety. Before an interview for a job or an examination there is a degree of anxiety. These feelings are all normal and they can even be beneficial because they prime the fight-or-flight response that improves how we carry out the task in hand. For more on the normal/abnormal distinction, see Chapter 4.

The symptoms of anxiety are both emotional and physical; they are listed below.

Symptoms of anxiety

Emotional symptoms	Physical symptoms
• Fear	• Stomach churning
• Tension	• Tense muscles
• Dread	• Sweating
• Uneasiness	• Flutter in the chest
• Excessive worrying	• Tremor
• Over-thinking	• Difficulty breathing

- Feeling disconnected from your own body (depersonalisation) or from things around you (derealisation)
- Feeling overwhelmed
- Low mood

- Appetite change
- Dry mouth
- Impaired sleep
- Rapid speech

The severity of the symptoms, their impact on how we function, and the nature of the event to which they are a response will determine whether we have a recognised psychiatric disorder or not. The anxiety that follows a stressful event in our life is discussed in Chapter 4. When there is no obvious trigger, or when the symptoms continue after the trigger has gone, a primary anxiety disorder can be diagnosed.

HOW MANY ANXIETY AND FEAR-RELATED DISORDERS ARE THERE?

There are five conditions in the anxiety and fear-related group:
1. Generalised anxiety disorder (GAD)
2. Panic disorder, with or without agoraphobia
3. Phobias
4. Social anxiety disorder (social phobia)
5. Separation anxiety disorder

1. Generalised anxiety disorder

Generalised anxiety disorder (GAD) is the term used to describe a *general* feeling of fear, that is, one without any specific focus. The person with GAD feels anxious for no reason. They will tell others that they do not know what they are anxious or worried about or, if there is some issue, their worry will be greatly in excess of its gravity. The symptoms of GAD consist of various combinations of those listed in box 5.1, but the *dominant* feature is a general feeling of tension. The experience is unpleasant. The person who is anxious may also feel depressed at times, but this is usually a consequence of the GAD, as this is of course very disagreeable. Anxiety can occur in most psychiatric conditions and, in particular when anxiety symptoms occur for the first time in those over the age of 40, this might indicate an underlying depressive illness, which would then be the primary diagnosis, rather than GAD.

Case Vignette

Ms A, a 30-year-old teacher, enjoyed her work. She had a particularly difficult class and had begun to worry that she might not be able to meet the demands they made of her. Her principal told her that she asked her to take this class because she was such a good teacher. She found that she couldn't relax even when she was away from school and her sleep was reduced; she found herself taking two hours to get to sleep. She was very preoccupied by the 'problem' of her class. She did not experience panic, but going to school was 'getting her down'.

Comment:
The symptoms in the example are typical of those seen in GAD. There are psychological and some physical symptoms. Worry is the dominant symptom. Her low mood seems to be secondary to her worry. She would benefit from psychological input. Cognitive therapy would focus on her preoccupation with something that is probably outside her control, i.e. the type of class. Learning to distance herself from a problem that she did not create and focusing on the very high standards she sets herself would be helpful. Mindfulness would be beneficial.

Note: This is not a real case but based on the features of many cases that the author has treated.

2. Panic Disorder

Panic disorder is diagnosed when panic attacks occur unpredictably. Usually there is a sudden onset of palpitations (heart thumping), combined with an extreme feeling of fear, chest pain, dizziness, sweating, and a fear of dying, collapsing, losing control or going mad. They may at times be preceded by a feeling of uneasiness. Overall there is a rush of some of the physical symptoms listed on pp.77-78 and the person feels the urge to exit their situation to relieve symptoms. Because of the intensity of the experience some (but not all) become fearful of places that induce panic and make them feel trapped or helpless. This progresses to agoraphobia (fear of public spaces either in or out of doors).

3. Specific Phobia

A specific phobia is a marked fear that is out of proportion to the danger, that occurs upon the anticipation of, or exposure to, specific situations or objects. These may be heights, certain animals, spiders, blood, lifts and so on. A phobia of cars or driving may follow a minor road traffic accident. The phobia is associated with avoidance of the feared object or situation, although some people may be able to endure exposure; even then, though, the exposure will cause intense anxiety.

Most phobias begin at a young age and certainly before the age of 40, except in very exceptional circumstances, and they affect the person's life to the extent that they hinder their occupation or their social, personal or educational life.

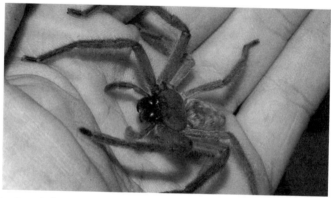

Arachnophobia is an intense and irrational fear of spiders and other arachnids such as scorpions. Treatment is typically by exposure therapy, where the person is presented with pictures of spiders or the spiders themselves.

4. Social anxiety disorder

Social anxiety disorder is more than shyness. It occurs when there is an excessive fear of social situations such as social gatherings (including conversations), being observed in the presence of others (especially eating or drinking), or performing in front of others (e.g. giving a presentation at work). The person is overly fearful that their actions will be viewed negatively by others. Social situations are avoided and this can result in isolation and loneliness. Social events such as eating in public, queuing and speaking on the telephone can prove very difficult and are even avoided. The impact on employment is significant if the person has to do presentations or chair meetings. It begins at a young age and there is often difficulty making friends even in childhood.

5. Adult separation anxiety disorder

Adult separation anxiety disorder most commonly occurs in children but it can afflict adults too. It is an abnormal fear that something bad will happen to a loved one, e.g. a fear that their adult child will leave home and never make contact or that a spouse will find somebody nicer than they are. The anxiety level may be high when they are away from their loved ones, e.g. if their spouse is away visiting another family member. Separation anxiety can also be directed to pets. The impact of separation anxiety is such that sleep and concentration may be reduced, and nightmares about the dreaded loss are common. Other anxiety symptoms are also present, and day-to-day functioning is impaired. The fears may circle around specific scenarios, such as abduction, fatal accidents or serious illness. This syndrome has only been recently identified in adults, and it is therefore seldom diagnosed.

HOW COMMON ARE ANXIETY DISORDERS?

It is difficult to be precise about how common anxiety disorders are because variations in their prevalence have been recorded around the globe. This is because of differences in the cultural attitudes to mental illness (which make it difficult to admit to problems in the first place), differences in how psychiatric disorders are expressed in various cultures, and differences in the questionnaires used to measure it. A ballpark figure suggests that 7.3% of the global population have a current anxiety disorder, though this figure could well be as low as 4.8% or as high as 10.9%, depending on which country the study is conducted in (Stein et al., 2017). They are more common among women than men. It is estimated that between 2% and 4% of the adult population has GAD at any one time and it is more common in developed than in developing economies.

Specific phobias tend to have an onset in childhood, social anxiety disorder usually begins in adolescence or early adulthood, and GAD, panic disorder and agoraphobia all typically have a somewhat later onset. Separation anxiety disorder was thought to occur only in children, but recent research suggests that it may continue into adulthood, or in some instances even have its *onset* then.

WHAT ARE THE CAUSES OF ANXIETY DISORDERS?

There are multiple causes of anxiety disorders. The personality of the person may place them at risk. For instance, someone who is of nervous disposition will be more prone to this sort of disorder. The trait of neuroticism (a tendency to worry about trivial matters) has been linked to these conditions. It is also likely that biological factors are involved, and indeed there is evidence that there may be a genetic predisposition to panic disorder and GAD at least (Morris-Rosenthal, 2002). Attention has focussed on gamma-amino-butyric acid (GABA), dopamine and serotonin, neurotransmitters that pass messages along the nerve pathways that determine our emotions.

HOW CAN ANXIETY DISORDERS BE TREATED?

There are two primary treatments for anxiety disorders: psychological treatments and pharmaceutical treatments.

1. Psychological treatments play a large part in treating all anxiety disorders. Generic counselling may help if the trigger to the symptoms is a particular problem. If the symptoms are more deeply rooted, CBT can help change one's thinking so that the anxious thoughts no longer fuel the anxiety symptoms. This is the most commonly used psychological treatment. For phobias, CBT can be combined with *exposure therapy*: this is a form of therapy in which the person meets the feared object either in their thoughts or in real time. This is done in a gradual and controlled way and, if successful, the anxiety lessens at each step. Social anxiety disorder is also best managed in this way, although two antidepressant drugs, sertraline and paroxetine, can also be effective at treating this. CBT

may assist in changing the fear of loss that is prominent in adult separation disorder, but sometimes a more psychodynamic approach that explores the origin of the fear, perhaps stemming from a loss in childhood, may also help.

Progressive relaxation exercises, in which different muscle groups are systematically tightened and then relaxed, are helpful for all anxiety disorders. They should be done once or twice each day and at a time when you are not rushed. Mindfulness, a therapy that draws on meditation techniques, helps you to focus on what you are sensing and feeling at the time. It is possible to train oneself in the use of these very helpful tools, but it is best, and easiest, to do so under some type of supervision until you are confident that you are doing them correctly.

2. For those with generalised anxiety or panic disorder, medications such as propranolol (also known as beta-blockers), are used to control the physical symptoms of rapid heart rate and tremor. These reduce the physical symptoms of anxiety but not the *psychic* (mental) anxiety. Pregabalin, also used for pain and for epilepsy, is used in GAD and panic disorder, as are the SSRI (e.g. sertraline), SNRI (e.g. venlafaxine) and tricyclic (e.g. dothiepin) antidepressants. These reduce both the physical and psychic anxiety. Benzodiazepines (e.g. diazepam) are also used for short-term help, but their long-term regular use is not recommended as they are addictive. If there are prominent anxiety symptoms when a person has adult separation anxiety, medication may be used to control the physical symptoms, while the underlying psychological need, of which the symptoms are the expression, is explored with talking therapy.

ANXIETY SYMPTOMS IN OTHER CONDITIONS

Anxiety symptoms can be present in most psychiatric disorders, but rarely are they the *primary* diagnosis. When anxiety accompanies another condition, the treatment of the primary condition should automatically lead to improvement in or the disappearance of the anxiety symptoms. This said, short-term use of antianxiety drugs may be necessary at times.

Other conditions in which anxiety symptoms are common

- Major depression/depressive episode (see Chapter 7)
- PTSD (see Chapter 4)
- Obsessive-compulsive disorder (OCD) (see Chapter 6)
- Psychosis (see Chapter 8)
- Normal responses to stressful situations (see Chapter 4)
- Thyrotoxicosis – overactive thyroid gland
- Pheochromocytoma – a rare tumour of the adrenal glands

DO PEOPLE RECOVER FROM ANXIETY DISORDERS?

With treatment, most people recover from anxiety disorders. Medications are usually only a short-term solution. Psychological interventions are very helpful but they have to be used regularly and the response takes several weeks. If the person is by nature anxious and has a tendency to fret over small things, the anxiety symptoms may take longer to control. In that instance the person may need additional help building self-confidence and learning to prevent ordinary day-to-day worries from getting out of control.

 ## WHAT YOU CAN DO FOR YOURSELF AND WHAT OTHERS CAN DO FOR YOU

- Seek help from your GP in the first instance.
- Use the multitude of online resources that are available (see p.85).
- Do not self-medicate as you may unwittingly become dependent, develop side effects or experience an interaction with other medication you are taking.
- Join a support group (see p.85).
- Cut out high-caffeine drinks.
- Avoid using alcohol or illicit drugs to relieve symptoms.
- Exercise.
- Try to gradually face the feared situation.

BIBLIOGRAPHY

Morris-Rosenthal, D. J. 'Are there anxious genes?' *Dialogues in Clinical Neuroscience.* 4,3. 251–60. 2002.

Stein, Dan, Scott, Kate M., de Jonge, Peter et al. *Dialogues in Clinical Neuroscience.* 19,2. 127–38. 2017.

USEFUL RESOURCES

Barry, Harry. *Anxiety and Panic: How to Reshape Your Anxious Mind and Brain.* London: Orion Publishing. 2016.

Butler, Gillian. *Overcoming Social Anxiety and Shyness: a self-help guide to using cognitive behavioural therapy techiques.* New York, NY: Basic Books, 2008.

O'Morain, Padraig. *Mindfulness for Worriers: Overcome Everyday Stress and Anxiety.* London: Yellow Kite/Hodder & Stoughton. 2015.

Williams, Chris. *Overcoming Anxiety, Stress and Panic: a five areas approach*, 3rd edition. London: Hodder Arnold. 2010.

'Progressive Muscle Relaxation Training'. Mark Connelly. YouTube.

'Guided Mindfulness Meditation on Overcoming Anxiety and Fear'. YouTube. 22 March 2014.

'Is Social Anxiety Getting you Down?' Lecture by Odhran McCarthy for Aware. YouTube.

National Phobics Society, Manchester. www.phobics-society.org.uk email: info@ phobics-society.org.uk

Social Anxiety Ireland, 8 New Cabra Road, Phibsborough, Dublin 7, and socialanxietyireland.com > getintouch

6

Obsessive-Compulsive Disorder

Obsessive-compulsive disorder (OCD) was first described as 'scrupulosity' in religious texts around six centuries ago. In the 15th century a Dominican friar, Antoninus of Florence, described scrupulosity as being caused either by the devil or as having physical causes. He described afflicted people as being 'smitten' with urges to constantly pray and forgive themselves. The 14/15th-century theologian Jean Charlier de Gerson recommended that the best approach was to ignore these urges. This may have been the first evidence of what we now call 'mindfulness', in which the person is encouraged to accept their symptoms. It was many more centuries, however, before OCD as we know it began to be diagnosed. In 1895, the term 'obsessive neurosis' was coined by Sigmund Freud, who described it as a defence against unacceptable ideas relating to sex and violence entering conscious awareness. The terminology and the meaning of the symptoms gradually changed, and by the 1970s, under the influence of behaviourism and cognitive theory, the modern diagnosis of obsessive-compulsive disorder (OCD) was born. In addition, developments in the neurosciences led to changes in the understanding of and approach to treatment of OCD so that it is now firmly founded on a medical and behavioural model. This is reflected in the treatments offered and in people's favourable response to treatment.

TERMINOLOGY

The word 'obsessive' is part of everyday language. We should be careful how we use the terms 'obsessional' or 'obsessive' because we also often speak of being 'obsessed' by something or somebody, such as a rock star or a TV programme. What we mean in this context is that we have a have a strong liking or preoccupation with the person or issue. This is normal and healthy, but it is very different from the powerful, repetitious thoughts and/or images that affect someone with OCD. As somebody once said to me when trying to describe his obsessional ruminations (see below), 'It's like a cine camera that's stuck'. Within OCD, those who are paralysed by the repetitiveness of their obsessional behaviour, such as spending long periods checking doors or washing their hands until they become excoriated, differ immeasurably from people with mild OCD habits, such as returning to check that the door is locked when you have a niggling doubt but deep down know it is fine, or from the healthy rituals seen in children who play hopscotch between the lines on paving slabs.

HOW COMMON IS OCD?

Around 1-2% of the population have OCD at any one time, but over a lifetime the prevalence is about 2.3%. It normally begins in the teenage years or early 20s, and comes and goes thereafter. Prior to the advent of the SSRI antidepressants and cognitive therapy, treatment options were limited and it was an extraordinarily debilitating condition that waxed and waned.

A related condition, known as obsessional compulsive personality disorder (OCPD), or anankastic personality disorder, describes those who in their psychological make-up are rigid, austere, perfectionistic and overly focused on order and rules. They are hardworking, but their perfectionism and rigidity make them unpopular with workmates and, most importantly, their behaviour causes problems with family and friends. It also has to be said that some large organisations may value this attention to detail and praise such people for their diligence etc., but close associates find them impossible to deal with them. OCPD affects between 2% and 7% of the population, making it the most common personality disorder (see Chapter 10). It becomes noticeable in the teenage years and remains with the person throughout their life. It differs from OCD in that the rituals and ruminations of the former are not present in OCPD. Those with OCD are often horrified by their ruminations and rituals. They see them as a problem and try to resist them. By contrast, those with OCPD normally see their traits as moral and proper and view themselves as more righteous than others.

It used to be the view that OCPD increased the risk of developing OCD, but recent evidence has now made the relationship more uncertain.

TELL ME MORE ABOUT THE SYMPTOMS OF OCD

Obsessive-compulsive disorder consists of two broad groups of symptoms: obsessional ruminations and obsessional compulsions (National Institute of Mental Health, 2019).

1. Ruminations are repetitive thoughts, ideas, images or impulses that continually intrude upon and enter the person's mind. The sufferer experiences these as very distressing because they know they are abnormal. In the early stages of the condition they try to suppress them, but this fades with time because of the sheer mental and emotional effort involved, and because it is not successful. As such, encouraging the person to put such thoughts out of their mind is an utterly futile exercise. Some say that accepting the thoughts, despite not wanting them, is a better first aid approach, as recommended by de Gerson (see p.87). The thoughts in OCD consist of repetitive deliberations about a variety of topics. These typically include numbers, the meaning of life, and phrases or ideas. Ruminations are of a different quality from thoughts as they focus on themes that enter the person's mind without any provocation (such as mathematical and philosophical thoughts). Sometimes thoughts about suicide enter the person's mind. A person with these thoughts does not want to die by suicide but the thoughts come to them unprovoked and there are problems supressing them despite their being unwanted. Unlike worries, which tend to be general (Will I get the job?), the equivalent in ruminations might focus on dress code being considered over and

over to the last detail of the actual clothes the person will wear. People with ruminations describe how wearisome they are and the utter exhaustion they feel.

Those who suffer with obsessional rumination are often ashamed of their content. It may be of a sexual, violent or blasphemous nature, even though these thoughts are unwelcome. Patients often think they are 'going mad', or that the content of the thoughts reveals something about themselves – such as that they 'really' want to hurt people or curse God. For these reasons, people are reluctant to consult their GPs or to tell others about them. However, it is important to stress that these concerns about consultation are unfounded. The intrusive thoughts of OCD are *not* your 'real' thoughts, and they do not mean that you are going mad.

2. Obsessive compulsions refer to compulsions to carry out certain actions. Compulsions are more common than ruminations and are clearly visible. A rumination, or even just a simple thought, may translate into behaviour, particularly where contamination is concerned, resulting in repetitive behaviour.

Common compulsive behaviours

| Cleaning | Avoiding | Repeating | Checking |

The person who has to return home to check that they have locked their front door 20 times, even though they know they have done so, is displaying a compulsive ritual. The person fearful of contamination may spend an hour in the bathroom, continuously showering or washing. They may refuse to touch door handles, money or staircases for the same reason. These repetitive rituals slow the person down in their day-to-day living. This is called obsessional slowness and can cause employment and family problems. For instance, if a person with OCD spends an entire hour showering this will impact on those they live with and will affect their work if, for example, they are constantly late. The range of compulsive behaviours is legion, from having to check and recheck windows, to exiting the car in a particular manner, to walking 10 steps forward followed by one step backward, to avoidance of buildings or clothing of a particular colour.

OCD is now regarded as a psychiatric condition grounded in a medical/behavioural model, largely as a result of developments in neuro-imaging studies. These studies have found a decrease in size in certain areas of the brain. It is not certain which neurochemicals are involved, but the fact that drugs that increase serotonin also improve the condition suggests that this system may be involved. In addition, about one third of first-degree relatives of those with OCD themselves have the condition, pointing to a genetic element.

VARIANTS OF OCD

A variant of OCD is trichotillomania, also known as hair pulling. It may cause people to pull their hair out at the scalp, the arms, eyelashes or any other site with hair. There is often a build-up of tension beforehand, followed by a reduction after the event. Sometimes the person is not even aware that they are doing this. There may be associated feelings of guilt afterwards. Bald patches may lead to low self-esteem due to embarrassment. Picking of the skin is called dermatillomania. This can cause bruising and bleeding and will sometimes leave permanent scars. Like trichotillomania, it too relieves tension.

Hoarding disorder (HD) is a recently recognised condition that is diagnosed when an individual has trouble getting rid of possessions that are no longer in use. Most of us from time to time are reluctant to dispose of certain possessions, such as those belonging to a recently deceased loved one or something to which we have a sentimental attachment, perhaps from childhood. This is normal and healthy. HD, by contrast, is constant, and the items hoarded have no special meaning or significance. The result is that the person's living space becomes almost unusable due to clutter and attempts to remove the items leads to significant anxiety. On occasion it can lead to eviction due to the fire hazard and other health risks it poses.

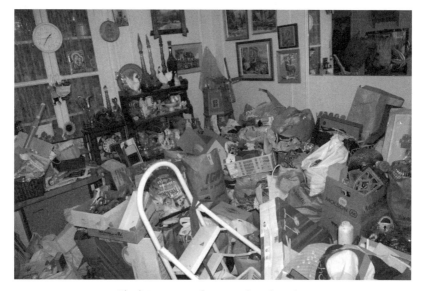

The living room of a compulsive hoarder

Obsessional fear of illnesses is another variant in the obsessional spectrum. It is also known as illness or health anxiety. To some it is known as hypochondria (see Chapter 13).

RESEMBLANCE TO OTHER SYMPTOMS

Sometimes it can be difficult to distinguish obsessional ruminations of OCD from one of the symptoms of schizophrenia (see Chapter 8), known as *thought insertion*. The key difference is whether the person sees the thoughts as their own or not. The person with OCD is aware that the thoughts are their own thoughts, although they find them distressing, whereas in schizophrenia, when thought insertion is present, the person believes that the thoughts come from some outside force, and are not the person's own.

OTHER CAUSES OF OBSESSIONAL SYMPTOMS

Obsessional symptoms can be part of depressive illness, and in that context the focus is on treating the underlying depressive episode.

TREATMENT

OCD is treated with a combination of medication and psychological interventions. Medications used are the SSRI antidepressants. One of the older tricyclics, clomipramine, is also effective.

Cognitive therapy in OCD exposes the person to the situation that is feared or encourages them to live with their distressing ideas and images. In mild to moderately severe OCD psychological interventions may work on their own, but often a combination of treatments is required, as this condition is *relapsing*, meaning that it will return if medication is discontinued. For many people, OCD treatment is a lifelong treatment, although once the symptoms are controlled, there is no reason why the person should not live a full, healthy and happy life. With continuing medication and psychological therapy, it has a very good prognosis.

Trichotillomania and dermatillomania are treated similarly to OCD.CBT is the favoured approach in hoarding disorder, with good results. Therapy focuses on reducing the acquisition of items while help in sorting and discarding objects is central too. The SSRI group of medications (e.g. paroxetine) or the SNRI group (e.g. venlafaxine) have also shown benefits.

 ## WHAT YOU CAN DO FOR YOURSELF AND WHAT OTHERS CAN DO FOR YOU

- Face up to your unwanted thoughts – you are not going mad.
- Face your fears, e.g. contamination.
- Persist in the above tasks.
- Read self-help books on OCD.
- Seek professional help if your self-help efforts are not successful or if you can't even begin them because of your distress.

BIBLIOGRAPHY

The National Institute of Mental Health Information Resource Centre. *Obsessive-compulsive disorder*. 2019 (online).

USEFUL RESOURCES

Veale, David, and Willson, Rob. *Overcoming Obsessive-compulsive Disorder: A self-help Guide Using Cognitive Behavioural Techniques.* London: Constable & Robinson. 2005.

https://www.rcpsych.ac.uk/mental-health/parents-and-young-people/ young-people/ocd-young-people

'OCD Treatment: Introduction to Exposure and Response Prevention (ERP)'. Katie d'Ath. YouTube. 16 October 2013.

'OCD Treatment: How to stop the thoughts! Katie d'Ath'. YouTube. 17 October 2013.

Thoughts out of control

———

Do you fancy her? Are you secretly gay? You're living a lie. Did you have a sensation there? God I don't think so. But what if it was sexual arousal? Oh fuck. Remember that thought you had about friends and family? Yes. Oh no. You're disgusting. Do I fancy them? Probably. Oh my god. I know I don't want to be with them. But why do these thoughts keep coming? Oh god here's another one ...

I initially thought I could solve these mental puzzles. I believed that I could control these thoughts. I believed that these thoughts were a manifestation of the 'true' me. I would embark on a mental quest to prove or disprove each idea. This was obsessive compulsive disorder (OCD), only I didn't know it then.

I first experienced intrusive sexual thoughts when I was 12 years old. I would get intrusive homosexual thoughts, images, sensations. I would be terrified by them. I would respond to every thought by trying to mentally solve, disprove, eliminate or neutralise them. These responses are actually compulsions only I didn't know that. Compulsions are anything you do to reduce the anxiety that the thoughts trigger. They seem to work initially but then a new thought comes along which causes anxiety and needs to be 'dealt' with. On and on it goes, cycle after cycle of panic and relief. Until you feel exhausted, drowning in doubt and removed from reality.

When I was not experiencing OCD I would look back at the thoughts and think, they're only thoughts, why was I so worried? I know who I am. I don't need to worry. All is well. Until the next episode of OCD. The same thoughts and images going round and round in my head. Causing what feel like mini heart attacks each time.

Then a new theme presented itself. Fear of infidelity. Why are my boyfriend and best friend getting on so well? Oh god look at them they just hugged. Oh my god what if he thinks she is more attractive than me? What if they kissed in the bathroom? I would never know. Oh god. Oh no. Round and round the terrifying thoughts would go.

Despite the mental torture I regularly endured, I had a great child-hood, teenage years and early adulthood. I had wonderful relationships with my family, friends and boyfriends. I also had success in education and enjoyed my many hobbies.

I went to my GP when I was 18. I told them that I was stressed all the time, I didn't tell them my thoughts because I feared they wouldn't understand. They might think 'she's gay and denying it' or 'she's a ho-mophobic asshole'. The GP recommended a psychologist whom I at-tended once a week for three years. I eventually told them everything. They said 'everyone gets thoughts like that, it's normal. Just let them in and out, they're only thoughts.' They weren't wrong but had no idea it was OCD and therefore didn't treat it. They misdiagnosed me with generalised anxiety disorder.

I had the most severe episode of OCD when I was on holiday with my family. The thoughts, images, sensations were endless. It was over-bearing. I wanted to die. I wanted to drown and never wake up. My mother knew something was very wrong. I spoke to my parents and they begged me to go to a psychiatrist. They had been suggesting it for years but I was reluctant to go. However, on this occasion I knew I had no choice – this illness would kill me if I didn't go.

I went to a psychiatrist a few days later. I remember sitting in their office and feeling relieved and safe. Here was someone who knew exactly what I meant, they understood all of the confusion and fear and torture that a part of my mind was causing me. Within 45 minutes of talking and listening to me they diagnosed me with OCD. It was as though I had been blind for years and someone gave me back my sight.

I did everything my psychiatrist recommended. I took medication every day and rarely missed a dose. I read the book they recommend-ed. I attended the OCD support group. All of this reduced the frequen-cy and intensity of my OCD by about 70%.

However, I wanted to be 90% OCD-free. At the recommendation of my psychiatrist, I went to a clinical psychologist to do Exposure Response Prevention Therapy (ERT). It involves deliberately thinking about the feared thoughts/ideas, images and sensations without engaging in compulsions, e.g. no 'checking' whether they are true or false, no 'reassurances' from self or others. A very important part of the therapy is to challenge fixed false beliefs and become comfortable with a lack of certainty. I did this for one year with an excellent psychologist. This improved my OCD by about 90%, as I had hoped.

I am very fortunate to have fantastic support structures in my wonderful family, boyfriend and close friends. Without them, I would have found it much harder to get to where I am today. I am currently working as a junior doctor, have great relationships with my loved ones and have a very good quality of life. I still have hard days with OCD but I can manage them much better now that I have a diagnosis, take medication daily and have ERT practice available to me.

7

Mood Disorders

Mood disorders are more than just everyday sadness. They are a group of conditions that do not fluctuate with the ups and downs of everyday life but have their own life independent of life's travails. Melancholia, a Latin term for 'deep sadness', was recognised by Hippocrates in the third century BC. He believed it resulted from an excess of black bile. This word is still used when describing certain symptoms that occur in depression, such as profound sadness, early morning wakening, feeling slowed up, worst in the morning, excessive guilt about minor issues. 'Depression' is the most common and most familiar of the mood disorders. Yet this is a loose term and most people who use the word do not in fact have any illness, because 'depression' describes a multitude of scenarios. They are summarised into six categories.

1. In day-to-day life people go through difficult patches. There may be a day that reminds them of better times gone by and they contrast this with their difficult situation now, or they may have a particular worry on their mind. The 'slings and arrows of life' are touching them and their mood is below par, but they will feel better when pleasant things happen. They might describe themselves as 'a bit down' or 'depressed'. This is not the clinical condition psychiatrists call 'depression'.

2. In many real-life situations, a depressed mood is appropriate. Indeed, its *absence*, not its presence, would indicate pathology. For instance, a person who has suffered the loss of a loved one will experience low mood as part of the grieving process. This will

last until acceptance of the loss is reached and the person begins to function again. Serious illness, the loss of a much-valued job, financial ruin, being bullied, domestic violence or assault can also cause sadness and a feeling of futility, or what we might loosely call 'depression'. The list is infinite. The mood change in these situations is often severe but because it is appropriate, it is not indicative of any illness and it lifts over time as the person adapts to their situation.

3. The use of certain substances – such as alcohol, cannabis and some commonly prescribed medicines like steroids, opiates, the contraceptive pill and antihypertensives – can lower one's mood. These are side effects that may require either stopping the drug, or a change in medication.

4. 'Depression' is also the term that is used to describe the clinical condition we call depressive illness, and this (properly called 'depressive episode' in ICD, or 'major depression' in DSM) is how I shall use the term in this book. It is the appropriate term used by doctors and mental health professionals. The restriction of the term to a clinical illness in mental health contexts is to avoid confusion with understandable low mood, and with the term as it is used in everyday language. Once an accurate diagnosis is confirmed, there are treatments available for depressive illness, both psychological and pharmacological, that are evidence-based and readily available. The illness is also associated with a certain symptom pattern that will be described further.

5. Depressed mood can occur as an inherent part of some conditions such as PTSD, schizophrenia etc. In these situations depressive illness is not the primary diagnosis but is *secondary* to the other primary condition. It may or may not require specific treatment in these instances.

6. Finally, some people with personality problems, such as emotionally unstable personality disorder exhibit rapid fluctuations in mood in response to very minor stressors. An argument with a friend will tip the person's mood, and the term 'depression'

is often inaccurately used to describe this mood instability. Antidepressants generally do not have any role in this condition, which is described in Chapter 10.

The focus of this chapter will be on depressive illness and its variants, including bipolar depression and dysthymia.

DEPRESSIVE EPISODE/MAJOR DEPRESSION

The terms 'depressive episode' and 'major depression' refer to the same condition, but 'depressive episode' is used in ICD, the WHO's diagnostic manual, while 'major depression' is used in DSM, the US diagnostic manual. The condition is said to affect about 5% of the population at any one time. Often the person is unaware they have it and attribute the symptoms to the weather, the absence of holidays, the menopause or any number of events. These things of course may indeed be responsible for how the person feels. The surest indication that the cause is depression is that the person's mood is *constantly* low, or that pleasant things give them a reprieve. If the low mood persists, and especially if there are other symptoms too (see below), then the person may have depressive illness.

Symptoms of depressive episode/major depression

Mild/Moderate Illness	Severe Illness
• Gloom/tearfulness	• Inability to cry
• Irritability	• Inability to feel
• Anorexia or over-eating	• Delusions[5] of guilt
• Anxiety: free-floating/panic attacks	• Delusions of persecution
	• Delusions of reference
• Agitation or retardation	• Auditory hallucinations, second-person critical
• Insomnia: early, middle or late	
• Hypersomnia (excessive sleeping)	• Nihilistic[6] delusions
	• Hypochondriacal delusions
• Aches or pains	• Delusions of poverty
• Depersonalisation[1]	

- Reduced concentration
- Lack of confidence
- Inability to cope
- Mood worst in morning
- Loss of interest, including sexual interest
- Overvalued ideas[2] of guilt, reference,[3] illness
- Obsessional rituals or ruminations[4]

See Appendix to this chapter for explanation of numbered symptoms.

Without treatment, depressive illness can last interminably. Before the availability of antidepressants severe cases often resolved spontaneously only to recur again, or were treated with ECT, as this was the only treatment available. Nowadays, the risk of depression recurring is around 25% within five years. If you require referral to a psychiatrist, normally because the episode is deemed to be of moderate or severe intensity and perhaps outside the GP's comfort zone, the chance of recurrence in the next five years is substantial, and over a lifetime is about 80%. So, the more severe the initial episode, the more likely the risk of recurrence. Unfortunately, for large numbers of people depressive illness is a recurring condition, but the good news is that this can be prevented in most people using long-term antidepressants (lithium), along with cognitive therapy.

HOW COMMON IS DEPRESSIVE ILLNESS?

The prevalence of depression at any one time in the general population in Western Europe and North America is around 5–8%, although there is some variation due to the methods used to gather the information. The lifetime risk is about 10% for men and 20% for women. In developed countries, the prevalence of depressive episodes increases from adolescence to age 25–35 years, then falls until age 60, and then increases again. Episodes in the elderly are generally more severe than in the younger age groups.

WHAT CAUSES DEPRESSIVE ILLNESS?

There is no single cause for depression. What we do know is that there are risk factors and protective factors. The prevalence is generally lower in working populations, among men, among those with third-level education, those who are married and those who are physically healthy. Other protective factors include having strong social supports, engaging in personal and community religious practice and not living alone.

Of the risk factors, the most noteworthy is that having a prior history or a family history of the condition increases the risk. The risk associated with a family history suggests that genetic factors are involved. This is not to imply that a family history will definitively result in a depressive illness. The likelihood is increased, but not inevitable, because protective factors also come into play. For instance, if someone with a non-identical twin suffers with this condition, the risk that their sibling will have it is about 28% (similar to the risk of a non-twin sibling having it). For an *identical* twin, the risk to the co-twin is 50%; when both parents have the condition, there is a three- to fourfold increase in the risk of depressive illness in their offspring compared to the general population.

Other risk factors are the trait of 'neuroticism' and childhood adversity such as separation from parents, abuse (sexual or physical), neglect or significant bullying at school. Major life events may also trigger a depressive illness. People with depressive illness and their families are often surprised to learn that having had one episode of depression, there will still be a risk of future episodes, even without a trigger, because the first episode will have resulted in continuing microscopic brain changes.

WHAT HAPPENS IN THE BRAIN?

The brain consists of millions of neurones which pass messages between each other. A number of changes have been identified in the brain using various imaging techniques, but no single change to the brain has been identified. MRI scanning has helped identify changes to areas of the brain that include the prefrontal cortex, cingulate cortex, thalamus and hippocampus among those with depressive illness compared to healthy controls. Other studies suggest that certain circuits in the brain between these locations are altered. These are like the wiring systems in an electric circuit, with the connections between certain key locations being damaged. So far, four of these connections have been identified in major depression (Zhang et al., 2018), although much more research is needed to confirm this finding. Ultimately, it is likely that what is currently called depressive episode or major depression will turn out to be several different conditions, each with its own neurochemical and neuro-anatomical pattern.

Another theory relates depression to changes in the 'stress pathway' between the glands in the brain known as the pituitary gland and the hypothalamus; changes to the hormones released by this circuit have been found in depressive illness. The neurochemicals that have been identified as abnormal include noradrenaline, serotonin, dopamine and melatonin. The thyroid gland in the neck is also important, and it has been shown to be associated with depression when it is underactive and with anxiety when overactive. It remains to be seen if any of these areas of investigation will inform future treatments.

DYSTHYMIC DISORDER

This is a condition that most readers will not have heard of, although it is thought that 1.5% of the population suffer with it. Dysthymia is also called *persistent depressive disorder*, and it usually begins in early adulthood. The symptoms, although less severe than in major depression, often linger for two years or more. There may be periods when the symptoms increase and the threshold for full-blown depressive illness is reached; this is called 'double depression'. Dysthymia is an uncommon condition, but for the sufferer it is disabling and disheartening. Because of the symptoms of low mood, irritability, loss of interest, low self-esteem and low energy, all of which are of long standing, it has a significant impact on day-to-day functioning, although less so than other forms of depression. Moreover, precisely because it is not as dramatic as a full-blown depressive episode, it can be particularly insidious. If you are worried that you or a loved one are feeling generally down but don't consider it to be serious enough to count as 'real' depression, it is worth considering talking to a GP anyway, as dysthymic disorder may be the culprit.

SUBTYPES OF DEPRESSION

There are five recognised variants of major depression:

1. **Atypical depression** is diagnosed when the person sleeps excessively (hypersomnia) and their appetite increases, resulting in weight gain. It is accompanied by an increased sensitivity to how they are treated by others, irritability, anxiety and a feeling of being 'weighted down'. Treatment is similar to that of depression generally, using both cognitive approaches and pharmacotherapy. However, some have argued that atypical depression is best treated with the older group of antidepressants known as the MAOIs (monoamine oxidase inhibitors).

2. **Melancholic depression** is characterised by early morning wakening, with mood lowest in the morning (this is known as diurnal mood change), and by experiencing little change when pleasant things happen (known as loss of mood reactivity). This type of depression responds to most antidepressants, but antidepressants with sedative properties are best since they will help improve sleep quickly and will also reduce anxiety symptoms more speedily. ECT is rarely used nowadays, but in this group it may sometimes be required for a full treatment response to occur.

3. **Psychotic depression** is the term used for those with symptoms listed on p.99 under the 'severe illness' category. It is relatively uncommon and requires an antipsychotic as well as an antidepressant. ECT it is sometimes required to bring about improvement.

4. **Seasonal affective disorder (SAD)** is the term used for depressive episodes that occur exclusively during the winter months. The person with SAD may sleep to excess and, oddly, have a craving for chocolate. The cause of SAD is that the neurotransmitter melatonin, which is affected by sunlight, has been compromised. Treatment with antidepressants is required for the duration of the season; these can be discontinued at the end of the season. Psychological therapy is normally given in combination with the antidepressants. Treatment is also aided by 'light therapy'. This

involves the person sitting under a specialist 'SAD' lamp for about 30 minutes in the morning or even twice each day. The lamp accurately recreates the brightness and colour of the sun, 'tricking' the brain into thinking the days are brighter and longer than they are. There is a variety of commercially available clinically approved SAD lamps with different features. Walking during daytime in winter also helps.

5. **Reverse SAD** occurs when depressive episodes occur exclusively during the summer months and is very uncommon. It is unclear if melatonin is involved, but one theory is that people stay up too late and disrupt their normal sleep-wake cycle, resulting in depressive symptoms. Because of its rarity there is little research to act as a guide. The treatment is with antidepressants and psychological therapy.

DEPRESSION DURING LIFE EVENTS

Depression in pregnancy

Depression in pregnancy and in the post-natal period is common. Estimates vary greatly across studies. Around 12% of pregnant women in Ireland are at risk of depression in the first trimester, 14% in the second, and 17% in the third. Those under the age of 18, those in lower socio-economic groups, and those with previous pregnancies have the highest risk. Studies from other countries, such as Sweden (Shakeel et al., 2015), have found somewhat lower rates – except for ethnic minorities, among whom rates were much higher, particularly among those who had not integrated. A prior history is one of the biggest risk factors. However, although depressive illness is a danger throughout pregnancy, it peaks in the post-natal period. The symptoms are similar to those in other sorts of depression, with the main difference being that the focus tends to be on the woman's competence as a mother. Treatment is the same as for depression in general. During pregnancy women may be reluctant to take an antidepressant, and, indeed, there are no antidepressants licensed for use in pregnancy, so they should be avoided if at all possible. Many women forego antidepressants in favour of psychological treatments. Where antidepressants are necessary, escitalopram and sertraline are the most frequently used. Paroxetine is not used because it is reported as causing cardiac problems in the unborn baby. For those who are breastfeeding, sertraline is the preferred choice. However, the response of the person to prior antidepressants should also be taken into account in making this treatment decision.

Since there is clearly variability in the choice of antidepressant during and after pregnancy, it is important to discuss things with your GP or psychiatrist before embarking on treatment. Obtaining information from the drug company is also a good idea – your GP or psychiatrist can request this information. The risks and benefits can then be discussed. The golden rule is that the lowest dose to maintain well-being should be used. It should be borne in mind that although antidepressants have risks, so does depressive illness in pregnancy or in the post-natal period: it can adversely the baby's development both in the womb and afterwards, as well as impacting on the mother-baby relationship.

Sometimes, in severe illness, psychotic symptoms (puerperal psychosis) may occur, and these too relate to the baby; for instance, the mother may have delusions that the baby has some serious illness, or that the infant isn't hers or has been substituted. The risk among those with no history of mental illness is one in 1,000, but the risk increases in those with a prior history of psychosis or a family history. When psychotic symptoms are present, medical staff will do their utmost to ensure the safety of both the baby and the mother. Admission to hospital may be required, and treatment with antidepressants and antipsychotics will be administered if deemed appropriate.

Depression due to pregnancy loss

This may be either through stillbirth or perinatal death, miscarriage or following a termination of pregnancy. Stillbirth is heartbreaking, and it is tempting to assume that everybody who experiences this is going to develop a depressive illness. For most it is grief like no other, associated as it is with the joy of pregnancy and the anticipation of the new baby, only to be followed by the tragedy of loss. Most women cope with the loss with time, and require support from family and from friends as well as from others who have experienced a similar loss. Some may require a psychological intervention, and some may develop a full-blown depressive illness requiring treatment. It is crucial not to medicalise the grief and turn to interventions, either pharmacological or psychological, too early.

It is understandable to feel sad after a miscarriage but in some women it can tip into a depressive illness – especially if there is a prior history. Among those who have had an induced abortion, the initial response may be relief but can be followed by low mood thereafter. Ambivalence about terminating the pregnancy, coercion and being ethically opposed to abortion increase the risk, as does a previous history of depression. Treatment is as for depressive illness more generally, with antidepressants and/or psychological therapy and possibly religious/spiritual interventions comprising the standard course of treatment.

Depression and the menopause

There is a myth that the menopause heralds a period of depression among women. This has been shown to be mostly incorrect, although there is an increased risk in those who have a previous history of depression or who have had post-partum depression. Those who had premenstrual dysphoric mood disorder (premenstrual depression) are also at risk. The period of greatest risk is actually the time *before* the menopause. Any woman with low mood at this time should consider attending a doctor, since the hormone fluctuations that presage the menopause could alter her mood. The role of hormones in treating depressive illness at this time is a matter of some debate. Besides a hormonal explanation, another possibility is that this time in a woman's life may be associated with the family growing up and leaving home, as well as with other losses through death, so hormones may not provide the whole answer, or may even be a red herring. Antidepressants and/or psychological therapy should be considered if the depressive symptoms are severe enough.

CAN DEPRESSIVE ILLNESS BE MISDIAGNOSED?

Depressive illness can be missed in some situations and can be over-diagnosed in others. It may be missed as a diagnosis when anxiety symptoms are prominent. This may lead to depression being misdiagnosed as GAD (see Chapter 5). In older people, depressive illness may sometimes cause mild confusion, leading to a misdiagnosis of dementia. Indeed, the confusion that occurs due to the slowed-up thought processes in depression in any age group is referred to as *pseudodementia*.

If obsessional symptoms are prominent, the condition may be misdiagnosed as OCD.

The reverse can also happen, and a person experiencing a stressor-related problem (see Chapter 4) may be misdiagnosed as having a depressive illness when the appropriate diagnosis would be an adjustment disorder. So the possibility of over-diagnosis is very real in clinical practice and in research studies due to the confusion in terminology and also the methods used to evaluate it. In addition, those with physical illnesses such as thyroid gland dysfunction may be incorrectly diagnosed with depression. Last, but by no means least, normal sadness may be mistakenly misdiagnosed as depressive illness.

WHAT ARE THE TREATMENTS FOR DEPRESSIVE ILLNESS AND DYSTHYMIA?

The first thing to be emphasised is that depressive illness is, for the most part, a very treatable condition. Those who do not respond may have been misdiagnosed, or they may not have taken the medication as prescribed. Others may be abusing substances that lower mood, and have either not disclosed it to their doctor or have not been asked about it!

For dysthymic disorder, antidepressants are usually tried, but they are often only partially effective if used alone. Purely psychological therapies have been shown to be effective too, although somewhat less so than medication. The combination of both together appears to be the most likely to bring about improvement.

For mild and sometimes moderately severe depression, psychological treatments may be effective, otherwise antidepressants are required, in the first instance for six to 12 months. This might seem like a long time, and the patient may feel that they are able to wean themselves off them before this time. However, it is strongly advised to stick with them for the full duration; the reason for the long course is to reduce the risk of relapse. If relapse does occur, then treatment may need to be indefinite, particularly if symptoms are severe and impact upon the person's work and day-to-day life to a significant extent. Suicide is also an ever-present risk that has to be minimised by reducing the frequency and severity of relapses.

There are several major groups of antidepressants, listed below.

Antidepressant groups

- Tricyclic antidepressants (TCAs), e.g. amitryptiline
- Serotonin reuptake inhibitors (SSRIs), e.g. fluoxetine
- Monoamine oxidase inhibitors (MAOIs), e.g. phenelzine
- Serotonergic noradrenergic reuptake inhibitors (SNRIs), e.g. venlafaxine
- Noradrenergic-specific serotonergic antidepressants (NaSSAs), e.g. mirtazapine
- Melatonergic antidepressants, e.g. agomelatine
- Others, e.g. vortioxetine, trazodone

Antidepressants are started in low doses and then increased every few days or weeks depending on the medication. If, after an adequate dose and appropriate duration of treatment, the symptoms have still not improved, treatment should be changed and combining medications needs to be considered if there is still no response. Difficult depression such as this is known as *treatment-resistant depressive disorder*. This sort of depression is common: about 60% of people fail to show an adequate response to the first antidepressant.

Combinations that are used for treatment resistance include the addition of lithium (lithium augmentation) to the pre-existing medication. The use of mirtazapine and venlafaxine in combination also has some evidence of benefit. The addition of some antipsychotic medications, such as quetiapine and aripiprazole, may also boost the effect of the antidepressant (NICE Guidelines, 2017).

If antidepressants combined with antipsychotic agents do not bring about relief in severe depression, particularly if the person remains psychotic or has depressive psychosis, consideration should be given to ECT. This is used under general anaesthetic. Antidepressants must then be used to maintain progress and prevent relapse. ECT is seldom used nowadays and is available in only a few centres nationally.

For depressive illness, psychological treatment such as cognitive therapy, interpersonal therapy and mindfulness are very helpful. For those

with moderate to severe depression, a combination of talking therapies
and medication achieve the best outcomes.

BIPOLAR DISORDER

The condition now known as *bipolar disorder* was previously known as
'manic depressive illness'. In the 1980s the name was changed to bipolar
disorder so as to place greater emphasis on the emotional symptoms, and
also because the word 'manic' had become popularised with potentially
stigmatising connotations, e.g. 'manic Mondays', 'homicidal maniacs'.
It was first described by Emil Kraepelin, a German psychiatrist, towards
the end of the 19th century. He also distinguished it from the psychotic
condition now known as schizophrenia.

Under the new terminology, two types of this condition are recognised: bipolar 1 and bipolar 2. The differences are listed below.

Differences between bipolar 1 and 2 disorders

Bipolar 1 disorder	Bipolar 2 disorder
• Manic – psychotic symptoms • Significant effect on day-to-day functioning • Invariably requires inpatient treatment	• Hypomania – no psychotic symptoms • Some impact on day-to-day functioning • Can often be managed in the community

The speed of change between the 'poles' – i.e. between mania/hypo-
mania and depression – is also relevant, and *rapid cycling disorder* occurs
when a person experiences four or more episodes of mania/hypomania
or depression in in year. Sometimes the gap may be only a few days
between each pole of the disorder. Of those with the disorder, 10–20%
have the rapid cycling form.

CREATIVITY AND GENIUS

Bipolar disorder has been linked to creativity and genius, and this has
helped to reduce the stigma of this condition. For example, Mariah

Carey, Catherine Zeta Jones and psychiatrist Kay Redfield Jemison all suffered with it. Vincent Van Gogh also had the condition and ultimately died by suicide in a depressive phase.

HOW COMMON IS BIPOLAR DISORDER AND WHAT ARE ITS CAUSES?

Bipolar disorder is diagnosed in around 1% of the population as a whole, a similar proportion to schizophrenia. The prevalence of bipolar 2 is around 10%, and some claim that it may be under-diagnosed.

In terms of the causes, one of the risks is a genetic one. It is well recognised that bipolar disorder is more common in families in which the condition is present. If a parent or sibling has the condition, the risk that someone else in the family will have it rises to 8%. The risk is also higher in families with members who have depressive illness. No single gene has been established as causing this and multiple genes are thought to contribute.

Environmental factors such as childhood trauma are also associated with developing bipolar disorder, as are acute or chronic life stressors. There are no medical tests for bipolar disorder, and in some who have the disorder there are no apparent risk factors such as those discussed here.

HOW DO I KNOW IF I HAVE BIPOLAR DISORDER?

As indicated above, both depression and mania/hypomania are required to make a diagnosis of bipolar disorder. Depression, as we have seen, is common in the general population (at around 7%), so, of itself, this does not indicate who will develop bipolar disorder. The diagnosis can only be made once an episode of mania or hypomania has occurred, and this may not happen for some years after the individual experiences a depressive episode. Episodes of manic-like behaviour are also linked to misuse of drugs, particularly those that are illegal, such as cannabis, cocaine, ecstasy, LSD and amphetamines, but mania in these contexts does not indicate bipolar disorder. A doctor would instead diagnose the episode as *drug-induced psychosis*. In the absence of drug misuse, though, the occurrence of a manic or hypomanic episode *will* lead to a diagnosis of bipolar disorder.

WHAT DOES A MANIC EPISODE FEEL LIKE?

The descriptions of what people feel like are twofold. Some are exhilarated by the feelings of elation and happiness and for this reason resent medications that control the mood swings. Others feel absolutely terrible due to the irritability and anger they experience. Some may also be over-familiar and over-talkative, with their words tumbling out. This is known as *pressure of speech*. Additionally, the thread of their conversation may be vague and shifting, and listeners may find themselves unable to follow it. This arises because the manic person's thoughts are running rapidly through their mind. This is known as *flight of ideas*. Disinhibited behaviour and acting in uncharacteristic ways, such as being over-familiar with others, being sexually promiscuous, intruding upon others' space in conversations, or over-spending are also often described. The money is used not just to buy minor items that are unnecessary but may involve spending thousands of euro on expensive items such as cars or designer clothes; and this profligacy may be committed by those not at all normally given to such extravagance. Grandiose and persecutory delusions may also be present during manic episodes, resulting in confrontations with others.

The conventional wisdom is that those in a manic state enjoy being there. However, although this is certainly true for some, others are irritable while in this state and may even become aggressive. The irritability appears unprovoked and is typically directed at an individual who perhaps asks very simple questions that normally would not be met with any rancour. This is called *dysphoric mania.*

The manic person may sometimes have delusions that they are famous or connected to royalty, that they have a special message and mission in the world, or that they are being told by God to behave as they do. These are delusions, and a common symptom of mania. The activities associated with these may result in the person getting into trouble with the law.

Hypomania is a less severe form of mania in that there are no delusions, the person may be more mildly elevated or only mildly irritable, and their restlessness and overactivity is more containable and controllable. Their speech, whilst rapid, may be possible to contain. Admission to hospital may not be required and it can often be treated as an outpatient or by attending a day hospital.

HOW IS THE CONDITION TREATED DURING THE DEPRESSIVE PHASE?

During a depressive swing the treatment is usually with antidepressants, although in recent years concern has been expressed that the use of antidepressants may cause a switch to the opposite pole of the disorder (hypomania or mania) rather than actually helping. Nevertheless, many psychiatrists will treat the depressive phase in the usual way while closely monitoring the patient. Checks should also be made that mood stabiliser dosage and blood levels are optimised, and that levels of lithium (if used) are in the appropriate range. This requires checks 12 hours after taking lithium. In order for the checks to be properly informative, the patient must make sure to take their librium at the same time every night.

HOW IS MANIA TREATED?

During the acute phase of mania, hospitalisation is invariably required and treatment is with antipsychotic agents in order to reduce the delusions, the over-activity and the elation. Once this has been achieved, a mood stabiliser is introduced. Similarly, when a bipolar depressive episode occurs, a mood stabiliser must be considered.

LONG-TERM TREATMENT OF BIPOLAR DISORDER – GENERAL PRINCIPLES

Mood stabilisation is required to control the episodes of depression and elation that are inherent in bipolar disorders 1 and 2. Some psychiatrists recommend that a mood stabiliser should not be added after a first episode of hypomania, although other psychiatrists take the view that having had one episode, a second is likely. Clinical judgement regarding the impact the first episode has had on the person's day-to-day functioning will also influence that decision, and this is a matter the patient should discuss with their psychiatrist. So, if somebody lost their job as a result of the severity of the first episode of mania, there would be a case for considering a mood stabiliser at that point. The usual approach is to institute this treatment if there have been three or more episodes over a two-year period.

The mood stabiliser with the best evidence is lithium. Others include carbamazepine, lamotrigine and sodium valproate, but the latter should not be used during pregnancy as it is associated with significant foetal abnormalities. Both carbamazepine and sodium valproate are also used in epilepsy. Some of the antipsychotics that are used in the treatment of mania and hypomania also have mood-stabilising properties, including olanzapine, quetiapine, aripiprazole and risperidone, on their own or when added to a recognised mood stabiliser. Before commencing a mood stabiliser, some baseline blood tests are required to check renal, liver and thyroid function, as well as calcium levels and heart function. The particular tests vary with the medicine being used.

The treatment for established bipolar disorder, whether 1 or 2, is lifelong. This is because episodes can recur if treatment is discontinued. If for some reason medication has been discontinued, e.g. because of pregnancy, this should happen slowly rather than abruptly, as this can trigger a manic relapse. If someone taking treatment for bipolar disorder is considering getting pregnant, she should talk to her psychiatrist about how best to do this without risking relapse.

If untreated, bipolar disorder runs a reasonably predictable course. The gap between the depressive episodes becomes longer, while the interval between the manic episodes reduces.

COMMENCING AND MONITORING LONG-TERM TREATMENT

Once a a decision has been made to commence treatment with a mood stabiliser, this will need to be monitored closely from the beginning. This is rarely done by the GP so it will involve attending a regular outpatient clinic or a designated lithium clinic run by the multidisciplinary team.

Lithium

It is recommended that it be taken once per day rather than using the twice-daily preparation. This is to reduce the risk of renal damage, which is a complication of lithium therapy.

Before commencing lithium, the person should have renal function tests, thyroid function tests and serum calcium checked. In addition, if they have a heart condition, they should have an ECG and sometimes an echocardiogram. These should be monitored every six months thereafter, but lithium should be checked every three months.

Lithium levels are monitored because the level at which the person achieves mood stabilisation has been identified clearly from studies. Lithium should be taken at the same time each morning in order to facilitate monitoring 12 hours afterwards. Thus, taking it at 10.00 at night allows for it to be measured at 10.00 the following morning.

If the blood level is too high, vomiting, diarrhoea, tremors and muscle weakness may occur. Fits and kidney failure may occur with severe toxicity. If the person has any concern about their levels they should contact their GP or psychiatrist immediately.

Lamotrigine

Baseline blood tests are required before this medication is commenced. There is no requirement to monitor the blood levels unless it is thought that the levels are too high.

Lamotrigine is believed to be best for those who have mainly had depressive rather than manic episodes. It may cause a serious blood condition called Stevens-Johnson syndrome.

Sodium valproate and carbamazepine are also used as mood stabilisers. Blood levels of these are less important than they are for lithium, since the therapeutic response does not correlate with the blood level. The relevance of blood levels is to confirm that the person is taking the medication or to confirm toxicity.

Carbamazepine

Those on carbamazepine should have baseline blood tests. Thereafter white blood cells should be checked regularly. Blood levels of the drug are required only if toxicity is suspected. The therapeutic response in bipolar disorder does not depend on the blood level.

Sodium valproate
The requirement for blood tests is broadly the same as for carbamazepine.

When antipsychotics are used as mood stabilisers baseline bloods should measure serum lipids (fats), liver function, blood glucose and measures of weight, BMI and abdominal girth. These should be repeated after six months and then annually. Olanzepine is particularly likely to cause weight gain.

PSYCHOLOGICAL TREATMENTS

For bipolar disorder, psychological therapies are much less helpful for symptom control. However, psychoeducation may help with ensuring your adherence to treatment and with identifying whether you are at risk of an imminent relapse. During a depressive swing, cognitive and inter-personal interventions may help. Manic episodes are much less likely to be helped by psychological interventions due to the loss of insight, the significant impairment in concentration, and the excitement or irritabil-ity that occur during such episodes.

MIGHT BIPOLAR DISORDER BE MISTAKEN FOR SOME OTHER CONDITION?

Schizophrenia may resemble bipolar disorder, particularly when the person has delusions of grandeur and if there is excitement driven by the underlying illness. Sometimes the doctor may have to defer mak-ing a diagnosis until enough time has passed that they can make further observations.

Emotionally unstable personality disorder (see Chapter 10) is asso-ciated with mood instability, usually in response to minor life stressors. Fleeting psychotic symptoms can also occur. The symptoms are not as sustained as in bipolar disorder.

Drugs such as cannabis, LSD and cocaine can induce happiness, excite-ment and psychotic symptoms that closely resemble a manic episode. This usually settles quickly, once the drug has left the person's body. Therefore, tests for these drugs should be done when a person first presents to hospital.

OUTCOME

Most people with bipolar disorder who adhere to treatment can live normal lives. If relapses occur, these will inevitably impact on education, employment and relationships. Additionally, with inadequate treatment, there is a suicide risk. Recent research shows that without treatment or with inadequate treatment, up to 20% of those with depression end their lives by suicide. This is most likely during a depressive swing or when people have a combined state of mania and depression (dysphoric mania, discussed above). Lithium has been shown to be particularly effective at decreasing the risk of suicide.

Relapses of mood disorders are common; however, they are mostly due to non-adherence to medication, and to the abuse of alcohol and drugs. As such, sticking to the medication and refraining from drug abuse are some of the most important things a depressed person can do to keep themselves healthy and happy. People struck by mood disorders do rebuild their lives, although it can take time and patience. We should remember those people with bipolar disorder who have become successful despite the obstacle relapsing illness posed. People such as Mariah Carey, Frank Bruno, Francis Ford Coppola, Patricia Cornwell, Kay Redfield Jamison and many others in the annals of fame have all spoken publicly about their struggles with depressive disorders.

WHAT YOU CAN DO FOR YOURSELF AND WHAT OTHERS CAN DO FOR YOU

- Avoid illicit drugs.
- Avoid drinking alcohol to excess.
- Exercise.
- Ask others for feedback once your treatment is established.
- Adhere to your treatment.
- Try to identify, with the help of family and your psychiatrist, the early symptoms of relapse. These vary from person to person and have to be identified collaboratively.

- Accept advice when a friend/family member thinks you are unwell.
- Attend a support organisation.
- Do not tell your family member to 'snap out of it' – they cannot do this.
- Do not tell your family member how lucky they are to have a job/family etc. – they cannot see this in a depressed state and it will make them feel you are undermining the depth of their despair.

APPENDIX 2

[1] **Depersonalisation** – feeling cut off/detached/outside oneself

[2] **Overvalued idea** – an unreasonably held belief that is false and that the person can accept as false. These ideas are not as fixed as delusions but they do dominate the person's thoughts.

[3] **Ideas of reference** – ideas that they are being referred to on TV or the radio or in conversation, when they are not

[4] **Obsessional** – repetitive thoughts on a specific theme or repetitive actions, e.g. constant checking (see also Chapter 6)

[5] **Delusions** – a false and unshakeable belief not based on reality, the falseness of which the person cannot be persuaded of

[6] **Nihilistic delusion** – a delusional belief that some part of one's body has disappeared or that one is dead

BIBLIOGRAPHY

NICE Guidelines: Short Form 'Depression in Adults: treatment and management'. 2017.

Shakeel, Nilam, Eberhad-Gran, Malin, Sletner, Line et al. 'A prospective cohort study of depression in pregnancy, prevalence and risk factors in a multi-ethnic population'. *BMC Pregnancy and Childbirth*. 15. 2015.

Zhang, Fei-Fei, Peng, Wei, Sweeney, John A. et al. 'Brain structure alterations in depression: Psychoradiological evidence'. *CNS Neuroscience and Therapeutics*. 24,11. 994–1003. 2018.

USEFUL RESOURCES

https://www.rcpsych.ac.uk/mental-health/problems-disorders/postpartum-psychosis (a leaflet on post-partum depression).

AWARE 9 Upper Leeson Street, Dublin 4. 015240361. info@aware.ie or supportmail@aware.ie

Barry, Harry. *Flagging the Therapy: Pathways Out of Depression and Anxiety*. Dublin: Liberties Press. 2009.

Miklowitz, David J. *The Bipolar Disorder Survival Guide*, 3rd edition. New York, NY: Guilford Press. 2019.

Redfield Jamison, Kay. *Touches with Fire: Manic-Depressive Illness and the Artistic Temperament*. New York, NY: Simon and Schuster. 1993.

Redfield Jamison, Kay. *An Unquiet Mind: A Memoir of Moods and Madness*. New York, NY: Alfred A. Knopf Inc. 1995.

Walport, Lewis. *Malignant Sadness: The Anatomy of Depression*. London: Faber & Faber. 2019.

Bipolar disorder – there is always an answer, just ask the question

When I was eight I was asked 'What are the odds of a coin flip resulting in heads?'. Where is the coin being flipped? And is someone catching it? 'It doesn't matter, Ronan,' with a smirk. I went back to trying not to listen although I always hear. Flip a coin into space, it may never land. Far-fetched, yes, but a valid thought. Flip a coin onto a hard surface and it can land in its edge. Unlikely, yes, but I've seen it happen. Flip a coin and lose it forever, your results are still unknown. I still don't know the exact answer to this question, and it used to frustrate me that people were so certain the answer is 50/50.

Ten years later I was repeating my Leaving Cert year, for no discernible reason. The previous year I had gone up to higher level maths three weeks before the exam and took on a question that hadn't been taught for 20 years. I passed the exam even though I taught my teacher how to correct my mock exam as he hadn't taught the question before. Another teacher asked how I studied enough to pass. I replied, 'I read the book, then did the question,' and once again, like one hundred times before, I read the expression of disbelief on another teacher's face, then stormed off in anger before hearing a response.

A decade later, at 28, I no longer hold resentment for anyone but myself. I had been playing guitar for about five years along with song writing. This began to sprinkle happiness on my dark days. Although my depression was in full flight for a decade or more I was still too proud to let anyone in. My music became my true narrative.

A year previously, on my 27th birthday, I began to find my healthiest addiction – or so I thought. I read books in a single sitting, one after another. Philosophy, physics, anything. Not long after, this new addiction for knowledge began to impact my sleep drastically. Three or four days with no sleep, just waves of thought crashing together with no hope of rest without smoking weed.

At the time I was living in Toronto, Canada. Weed was legal but I over-indulged and it began to backfire. I became paranoid and reckless, which led to my diminishing rational thoughts. The depression enveloped me completely to the point where I entertained suicidal thoughts.

Now, with that being said, I never entertained those thoughts for too long. I read about the absurdity of suicide in Plato's *Phaedrus* and thankfully his words stayed with me. But I also have my family and friends to thank for my unwavering strength in the face of these over- encumbering thoughts. They are the sources of inspiration that I am profoundly lucky to draw from whenever it's needed. With this inspiration I have written some of my better songs and performed them for many people.

It's present day and I have just turned 32. I have been diagnosed with bipolar disorder. I had two separate visits to the psychiatric hospital. The first visit made feelings I had buried and ignored for years resurface. I was interviewed by many doctors, some of whom took notes labelling me delusional and grandiose. They didn't give me a fair analysis at first which brought back an anger I hadn't felt for years. I was prescribed a low dose of the tablets. I wanted a high dose of X and was prescribed an extra tablet, which did not agree with me. These tablets ruined my days for months. I could not think, I couldn't move purposefully, and I was socially anxious for the first time in my life.

A good friend who I have always trusted urged me to question the doctors on my medication until they dropped the second tablet. My personality came flooding back instantly but I still wasn't sleeping. The tablets I was on were not strong enough so I turned back to weed and in the beginning it worked. I got sleep and had a routine time happily until my tolerance went up. And eventually I was battling my greatest advisory once again, my mind.

One year ago, with my mind in turmoil once again, I had a conversation with a friend who asked me what it's like in my head. I said I don't have trains of thought, I have planes of thought, coming and going from my 'hairport' incessantly. He said, 'You are like a toddler in a Formula 1 car, you need to learn how to drive.'

Soon afterwards I went to my GP and he said I am the exception to the rule. At this point my confidence was high. My doctor and friends believed in my intellect, which was something I needed from an early age, but I never had it. My GP recommended me to go back to hospital, so I did.

This time I took everything I was told by doctors and nurses, and challenged their reasoning a lot, with the aim of increasing my desired medication and it worked. It was increased more than tenfold to the point where it actually calmed my mind and I could sleep soundly.

While I was in the hospital, I talked to many intellectual bipolar patients and realised I am not the only exception to the rule. Since I have got the right medication I am stable and productive, I have finally decided what I want to do with my life and that is to help people navigate their minds and believe.

Words are a key to success. The doctors and nurses in mental health have a monumental task in helping patients; they can only be successful if the patient is ready to open up. So if you are struggling, talk to someone. Ask for help and you will get it. Your life is worth living; no matter what you are going though there is always an answer. Just ask the question.

I am now in charge of my depression

Depression is not to the fore for me all the time. At times, I handle life well. I can be strong and resilient and life moves along smoothly. I can be productive and creative. If my mood drops I can rally and life gets back on track.

Nevertheless, when a serious depression sets in, life is different. For many years, I did not know or recognise I had depression. I thought my negative thoughts and feelings of inferiority were my own fault. I would often be angry at myself. I now know depression and I will give you some insight into my experience with depression. For me depression is a difficult word. It is a heavy word. It weighs me down. It pulls my heart down, just as surely as if a weight were attached. I feel disconnected from life. Nothing is interesting and nothing matters. Everything is tinged with a sense of loss or sadness. Depression is lonely. It is invisible. I am often not conscious of myself or of my needs. I feel trapped in a heavy fog and I cannot figure out or connect to what is going on around me.

I have always been prone to depression. However, my first major depression occurred with the sudden and unexpected death of my father when I was 19 years old. My world stopped turning. In the aftermath, I found it difficult to engage socially and I withdrew and isolated myself as much as possible. When I did engage, it took huge effort. It was exhausting keeping up the pretence of enjoyment. I saw my friends, laughing and chatting, but I felt myself separated and removed from time and space. My body was there but I was not. It was probably around this time that the natural curves of life's ups and downs morphed in a rigid straight line, where I felt no happiness and no sadness. I operated from a low mood base. I never spoke of the loss of my father for many years. I split from all emotion and feelings. I did not get close to anyone at this time and I let nobody close to me, for several years.

When a vague awareness crept into my mind that something was amiss I blamed myself for my predicament. I felt utter helplessness and despair. I could not make sense of myself. I had cut myself off from people, from life and from myself. I considered taking my life because I felt there was nothing left for me. I believed there was no coming back from this. I am unsure how I struggled through this time, but I did. I tried to figure out what I used to enjoy doing, what it was that made life meaningful. I did not know what was wrong with me, so I had no idea of where to seek help. I could see nothing worthwhile in myself. A chance encounter led me to take up a college place. I met new people. I was pleasantly surprised to find enjoyment in both the social and academic sides of study.

A physical health crisis in my mid-30s and a hospital admission brought a diagnosis of depression. I was shocked. I actually believed the diagnosis was incorrect. When I was discharged from hospital I headed straight to the bookshop to source some reading on depression. I began to understand for the first time in my life what had being going on within me. I recognised myself on every page. If (if if if if if) I had only known this sooner, I could have short-circuited years of sadness and distress. So to anybody who is reading this, your mental health is just as important as your physical health. They are viscerally connected.

When I became a mother, a second major depression set in. I was haunted by the belief that I was incapable of being a loving and caring mother. I feared I could not love my beautiful child. The pain of these feelings cut deeply into my psyche. I felt shame and guilt. I felt sorry for those around me who had to put up with me. I felt I could do nothing well enough. My heart was broken by the certain knowledge that my child had such a poor mother. The fact that my child was healthy and happy and that I managed the demands of domestic life and did my best, completely escaped me. I was unable to admit how I felt to anybody, let alone myself. However, this time, my depression did not continue for years. It was short-circuited because I did have professional help, and with medication and counselling returned to good mental health.

To be in charge of depression means that you need to learn what makes you tick, what sparks your motivation, and then, when you find it, bring that space or activity into your life. I know I need a creative outlet, I need to read and at times I need to go for a drive or cook with Leonard Cohen. It's the timbre of his voice and his words that work for me. I keep active and actively maintain friendships. I may not always be motivated to do tasks or to socialise, but if I encourage myself to make a start, I have found that the motivation often follows. Mindfulness has helped me to know, accept and like myself. A few minutes of turning inwards with kindness and gentleness keeps me grounded and connected to my thoughts and feelings.

Depression will remain present in my life. I continue to need medication, but I have built up the skills to recognise its reappearance and I seek the help I need. I am now in charge of my depression.

A successful treatment for bipolar disorder – medication and therapy

I am a 52-year-old man, living in Dublin, Ireland, who has lived with the mental illness known as bipolar disorder, or manic depression, all my life. I do not hate my condition, as it is an illness and I have learned to live with it. In fact, I have a love/hate relationship with my condition. When my illness is bad, it's very, very bad and when it's good, it's very, very good. It has shaped my life from my youngest years to the present day.

It unfortunately can be self-destructive and also extremely enjoyable, I have had my best moments in my life when I was high, I can be extremely creative when I am high or elated. I can write a script, or compose a bass line, or come up with a great award-winning idea for an advertising campaign for work. In fact, as a career I am paid to be creative, so it has its benefits.

Unfortunately when the high is over I come down with a bang, and slip in to the darkest of darkest depressions. I have been suicidal, stayed in bed for weeks – unmotivated to eat, to go outside or to meet friends, and I just want to lock myself away until the darkness passes. I have lost jobs due to my condition, I have wrecked relationships with past girlfriends by cheating on them or just being unbearable to live with. I have been promiscuous, even reckless.

When I am high I am the life and soul of the party, the 'cool' guy who can entertain you, make you laugh, be the best friend you've ever had. I will promise you the world and you will believe it all. I can walk into a bar and chat up the most attractive woman, without fear of consequence, without shyness or lack of confidence. I have slept with prostitutes, maxed out my credit cards, overdrawn my current account – and then I will wake up one day after going without sleep for weeks, a shivering wreck, asking myself, 'Oh my god, what have I done?'

There are no limits to the high when you are high, and there are no depths of depression I haven't experienced. I have been literally through hell and beyond and to heaven on earth. And, believe me, I am not comfortable in either place. I like to be in the middle zone, relaxed, calm and, as the doctors like to call it, 'stable'.

There is no easy way to describe what it's like to be high, but imagine your brain for a second, stuck in fifth gear, accelerating and getting faster all the time. Racing thoughts pulsing through your brain, at the speed of light. I describe it as like 'a fire in the brain' or 'bottled lightening' – and that's what it feels like, an electric charge firing non-stop – where every idea, every grandiose plan, every creative thought, must be acted upon without hesitation, must be written down and acted out. I have felt like the next Jesus Christ where I will save the world, a tycoon of the advertising world, a playboy, a poet and a rock star, or all of them combined!

Don't get me wrong, it feels great, but it won't last, you will isolate your friends, your family and loved ones. They do not know how to handle you and you will be completely oblivious to their warnings and concern. And then you will crash, and crash you will, and if you don't end up in hospital or get immediate treatment you can kill yourself from unemployment, shame, financial ruin, homelessness, self-loathing and utter despair. It's a very dangerous condition and it can be life threatening.

I have been hospitalised in the past, it's that serious. But It hasn't beaten me yet! And it never will. I have learned to live with it. I recognise the symptoms, of the highs especially, but the lows too. And you have to be vigilant for both. I know, for example, if I skip breakfast, stay in bed too long, and feel under-motivated, then I need to act. When I am getting high – if I ring everybody, talk too loud and talk too fast, I need to act. I recognise some of the triggers.

Over time and with the crucial assistance of my therapist, I have learned to recognise the triggers that send me into a high-elated state. They seem to have psychological connections to my childhood, and any bad memories related to my childhood are triggers, as well as any type of stress. It can be something as major as a death in the family or even somebody famous dying, but having to borrow money is a good example, especially from my mother. I hate asking for money, because I feel I am reverting back to my childhood, looking for help, and as a 50-year-old man that seems preposterous to me and shameful, and my pride is hurt. I do not want help! But ironically I need it. In fact, I probably would be dead from suicide due to excessive spending if I hadn't the love and support of my family and friends.

I am lucky, my mother and my family have bailed me out of financial ruin on so many occasions I should register as a bank. I hope you are as lucky as I am to have friends and family like them, a person/persons you can go to when life spins out of control. If you do find a friend, a loved one you can trust and who understands your situation, assure them it will only be a temporary situation. From time to time you will need help – and don't forget or be afraid to ask for help. Always ask for help when you need it – help is there 24 hours a day, through either helplines or mental health charities, and if it's an extreme episode of mania where you have been awake for hours and not taken any medication you are entering the danger zone, go to your doctor or ER at once. Go directly to hospital, do not pass Go and do not collect €200. Go now!

I take medication for my mood, 1000mg of sodium valporate daily to stabilise me, and usually 1mg of risperidone daily (and 2mg if I am particularly 'high'). The risperidone is my miracle drug. It kills the high in its tracks and has allowed me to hold on to my job as a successful graphic designer and art director and be financially stable. It has helped maintain my friendships and close relationships with my family. I have told my employer that I am bipolar. I was so relieved it was palpable. We discussed how we can reduce the stress which is a trigger and to communicate with each other when I am high. We have agreed that my boss will inform me if I am giddy, talking too much or overly excited and when I am generally being a pain in the ass! I also try to avoid alcohol as it dilutes the effects of the medication and this is not easy but I try.

To families and friends of bipolar sufferers, please stand by them and love them, even when they're out of control. They need you then, more than ever, and when they are at their lowest ebb and isolating themselves, keep calling and checking up on them. Keep the lines of communication open and call the ill person at least once a week.

To my fellow bipolar sufferers I say, 'Hang in there! Don't give up and stay alive!' You will get through the highs and the lows. Never ever consider taking your own life – no matter how bad you think your situation is or how much your mind tries to convince you to do it, don't do it! You are loved and cherished as a human being and you will survive it – it is a temporary setback and that's all it is. Temporary! Learn to live with your condition, recognise the triggers and take action at once, and keep talking to your doctor, family, friends and therapists – heed their advice and warnings and, most importantly, keep taking your meds! They will keep you alive.

Enjoy your life – you are not alone.

Finally, a word of thanks to the HSE and Pr C and her team at the M Hospital, Dublin, who have treated me so professionally over the years and taken care of me in my darkest hours. Thank you. I owe you my life.

Dedicated to my loving family, who have stood by me through the highs and the lows, the best and worst times.

– *Stephen G. Waller, 52, self-employed art director*

Living with bipolar disorder on my terms

———

I have a diagnosis of mental ill-health since 1998. I have struggled with my mental health to a greater or lesser degree both before and since then, with good periods of remission, and very significant periods of problematic symptoms.

When I was first diagnosed, it was bipolar I was diagnosed with, but that diagnosis has changed over time, and then one that sticks most often now is schizo-affective type disorder. At the time of my first diagnosis, I was living in America and working a responsible job that I loved; in a way, it was my 'dream' job, but it was the job that eventually led to my undoing, mentally.

In a sense, I was blinded to the fact that everything could go so wrong so quickly, and I was just lucky that I had enough insight that I could seek help immediately and ended up in the hospital instead of the morgue.

Abroad, I had few family supports. I was a young woman with a partner who had limited insight into what was going on and no experience of mental ill-health. We struggled dreadfully the first year and finally agreed to separate from each other. By that stage, I had long given up on my dream job, and could not see myself holding down another one for too long. My options were limited and closing in on me all the time. I arrived back in Ireland in May 1999 with just one suitcase and a backpack and immediately began to feel paranoid, something I hadn't remembered feeling before.

Like many returned immigrants with few housing options, I ended up in my mum's box room and slowly began to eke out a life and a living for myself with the help of my family. It was quite unfortunate for me that my mum had moved house since I had left for America, and I did not know well the area in which I was living, and most of my friends had moved on in their family lives and jobs.

Not to mention the stigma of mental ill-health that I felt, which brought me shame, and, of course, I might also have been in denial about the matter. But I was happy to have the roof over my head and the company that I needed at that time. Perhaps that makes me sound self-absorbed, but that is something that people with mental illnesses are accused of all the time.

In my experience, however, many times it is other people, and sometimes even well-meaning family members, who don't have self-experience of any disability, who lash out or show incredible lack of insight because they have not done any personal work on themselves to help them deal with their own issues, whatever they may be.

The conversation and dialogue around mental health are changing, and the media and interested lobby groups around mental health have contributed to that discussion. Still, it is often the person with self-experience of mental health problems that ends up excluded from their family, unfortunately.

I joined the Civil Service in 2001, and that was a great blessing for me in many ways, as it gave me great dignity at work, that I somehow felt that I didn't deserve or get in some of my dealings with other people or family members, especially after my mum died.

I got promoted at work after a couple of years and then again before the last recession. I felt respected and that the work that I was doing was valuable. It wasn't easy. During the periods of remission from ill health, when I took medication that worked and had talking therapies that were sort of satisfactory, it was fine, and life wasn't so much of a struggle. But there were times when my personal life would take over, and I would feel overwhelmed by my emotions, fears and thoughts.

Five years ago, my medication stopped working the way it used to, and I began to feel and behave oddly and impulsively in a way that I hadn't previously. I began to remember events that were so significant in their way, that I should have always remembered them, and yet they seemed like brand-new memories, even though the timeline was 20 or 30 years earlier.

I remembered many events and people from abroad, and to this day, I am not sure of the exact issues surrounding them or what the truth is regarding these. So, for that reason, I now describe myself as a person with a memory disorder, of sorts, coupled with the mood and psychosis element of my symptoms, which still manifest themselves occasionally.

I've had some difficulties and periods of great joy, sadness and many other emotions through the intervening years. I retired from work early a couple of years ago due to the difficulties in coping in the office. Now, I write for a magazine occasionally as well as study and write. I have self-published a couple of books since I retired.

As I write, I am now at home during the Covid-19 lockdown, and this has suited me to a certain extent because I don't feel the pressure to leave the house. I have a supportive partner who works from home, and I get a great deal of support from him. But I know I would be better off getting out and about and going for walks every day.

The comorbidities concerning additional medical problems for people with self-experience of mental ill health are always a concern for people with mental health problems, who may tend to suffer more with weight problems, diabetes and other risks for serious ill health. My fear for the future is that I will succumb to one or more of these problems, mindful of the fact that ordinary people with mental illnesses tend to have a shorter life expectancy for precisely these reasons. I would say that with all the medical care and therapies that I have got over the years, I now live life on my terms, and will have no regrets should that prove to be the case.

— CMK, November 2020

8

Schizophrenia and Other Psychoses

The *psychoses* are a group of conditions that are characterised by a loss of contact with reality. The list of psychotic disorders is as follows:

- Bipolar disorder (see Chapter 7)

- Depressive psychosis (see Chapter 7)

- Schizoaffective disorder

- Schizophrenia

- Delusional disorder

- Drug-induced psychosis

- Organic psychosis

- Micropsychosis (see Chapter 10)

HISTORICAL BACKGROUND TO SCHIZOPHRENIA

The term schizophrenia was first used in 1909. Prior to that, the condition was recognised, but it had a different name: 'dementia praecox', meaning a premature dementia. The term is not stable even now: some have argued that the term 'schizophrenia' should itself be abandoned and another diagnostic label found so as to reduce the stigma of the condition. This, however, is unlikely to happen.

HOW LIKELY AM I OR A MEMBER OF MY FAMILY TO GET THIS CONDITION?

The risk of developing schizophrenia over a lifetime is around 1%, and the number of new cases diagnosed each year (the disease's *incidence*) is between two 0.2 and 0.5 per 1,000 adults.

While schizophrenia is uncommon, it is the most serious of the psychiatric illnesses. This is because, without treatment, it can have a devastating effect. It affects the person's functioning in daily life and also causes great distress for their families. It was this group of patients in particular who, prior to the advent of medication, required longer-term hospitalisation because of their continuing symptoms, the deterioration in their day-to-day habits and functioning and the changes to their personality. Many remained there for the rest of their lives. With the discovery of drugs such as chlorpromazine in the 1950s in France, people with this condition began to experience symptomatic relief and even became well enough to be discharged home from hospitals. As a result, the notorious high walls of psychiatric hospitals were knocked down, their gates were opened, and ultimately the hospitals themselves were closed. In Ireland there are now very few psychiatric hospitals in use. Most have been transformed into hotels. People suffering from schizophrenia still require psychiatric hospital treatment, but this is now done in general hospitals, and the admissions are short term: days or weeks rather than years or lifetimes.

WHAT IS THE CAUSE OF SCHIZOPHRENIA?

There is no one cause of schizophrenia. However, drugs of abuse, such as cannabis, cocaine and amphetamines can trigger psychotic episodes, and in some these may continue even if the person no longer abuses these drugs (see Useful Resources, p.148)). So what began as a drug-induced psychosis now arises with no obvious cause; schizophrenia is diagnosed if the symptom pattern for that condition is present.

The importance of a genetic contribution has been recognised for several decades. Various genes have been investigated, but no single gene has been identified and there may be several genes that operate in combination. Evidence for a genetic contribution comes from the risk to a child who has relatives with the condition. These risks for different types of relationship are indicated below.

Risk of developing schizophrenia where a relative has the diagnosis

35% IF TWO PARENTS ARE AFFECTED

12% IF ONE PARENT IS AFFECTED

35-60% IF AN IDENTICAL TWIN IS AFFECTED

9-26% IF A NON-IDENTICAL TWIN IS AFFECTED

8% IF A SIBLING IS AFFECTED

2.5% IF A COUSIN IS AFFECTED

Older theories from the antipsychiatry school of psychiatry in the 1960s, of which R. D. Laing was probably the best known, suggested that it was the family environment that caused the condition we call schizophrenia. Another popular theory was called the 'double bind': according to this theory, schizophrenia arose from a disconnect between the verbal and non-verbal communication between the ill person and their parents in their day-to-day life. It was argued that schizophrenia was the only response to this situation. Other writers talked about the 'schizophrenogenic mother', who was both rejecting but also over-protective. The philosopher Michel Foucault saw psychiatry as one of the many institutions of coercion and discipline that contributed to the illness. None of these theories, however, was supported by research findings and they no longer have any clinical credence. They do, however, form part of the rich history of psychiatry and antipsychiatry that have made the specialty so invigorating to work in.

There is some evidence that the environment *contributes* to aspects of schizophrenia (Dean, 2005). Studies over the past 15 years suggest that living in an urban area is associated with an increased risk of developing schizophrenia and other psychoses. This, though, opens up another question: what is it about the urban environment that poses a higher risk than the rural one? Studies in migrant and ethnic minority groups suggest that the risk of schizophrenia is also substantially higher in first- and second-generation migrants, and similar questions are raised by this finding. Various explanations have been offered, including poverty, low access to healthcare, poor social supports, rates of illicit drug use and the social fragmentation of urban life. It was initially thought that the high rate of schizophrenia in cities was due to the movement of people with schizophrenia into the anonymity of city life, but recent studies suggest that it may instead be exposure to the urban environment during the child's upbringing that places them at risk of schizophrenia in later life. The mechanism by which this occurs, though, has not been established.

Other risk factors identified include obstetric complications and season of birth (winter and spring), due to an increase in infection. Elevated rates of cannabis use have also been linked to schizophrenia. Some have suggested that child sexual abuse is associated with the development of later psychotic symptoms, but others claim that the symptoms linked to abuse are less disturbing and less clear-cut than those usually found in schizophrenia.

Biological factors have also been implicated in the causation of schizophrenia. In particular, drugs of misuse may affect dopamine release, the neurochemical linked to schizophrenia. The role of stress, with its release of corticosteroids, has also been suggested, but the psychotic episodes triggered by intense stress last for short periods, generally less than one month. This is called acute and transient psychotic disorder.

Brain-imaging studies have confirmed that certain parts of the brain known as the lateral and third ventricles show enlargement in those with negative symptoms (see opposite). Other studies have found that the areas of the brain known as the hippocampus and amygdala are smaller, and some researchers have found overall differences in size between the right and left sides of the brain in those with schizophrenia and similar psychoses.

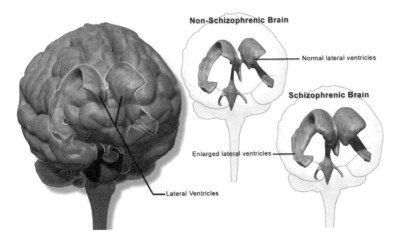

Non-Schizophrenic Brain

Normal lateral ventricles

Schizophrenic Brain

Enlarged lateral ventricles

Lateral Ventricles

Comparison between a non-schizophrenic brain and a schizophrenic brain

WHAT ARE THE SYMPTOMS OF SCHIZOPHRENIA?

The symptoms that indicate psychosis are hallucinations (seeing, hearing, smelling, tasting or feeling sensations, but without any stimulus to cause them) or delusions. So the person who has auditory hallucinations believes that they can hear somebody talking about them, yet when they turn around there is nobody there. The hallucinations are often speaking about the person and so use the third-person pronoun ('she/he') to refer to them. They may also give commands, and these are particularly worrying if they direct violence against oneself or others.

'Delusions' have a specific meaning in psychiatric contexts: they refer to *false, unshakeable* beliefs that are *out of context with the culture of the individual*. So, for instance, a belief in God is *not* a delusion, since even if this belief is false (which is a philosophical matter that is not for psychiatrists to decide), it is not 'out of context with the individual's culture': lots of people believe in God. By contrast, a firm, unshakeable belief in aliens landing on earth *is* a delusion: not only is it false, it is also out of context with the individual's culture.

Thought alienation is a specific type of delusion, one that relates to one's own thoughts. 'Alienated' thoughts, as they are known, are delusional beliefs that one is not in control of one's own thoughts, but that thoughts are being inserted, withdrawn or broadcast by some outside force. These experiences must refer to a specific thought rather than thoughts in general. So believing that our thinking is being controlled by what the media tell us is not a delusion – this belief is too general – but by contrast, believing that aliens caused one to have a thought last night about the end of the world *is* a delusion.

Beliefs that specific actions one engages in are being directly controlled by others are called *passivity phenomena*, and are also delusional. Again, specificity is important: a belief that governments are *generally* monitoring our activities, or that by their laws they are impacting on behaviour, is not a delusion. However, if a person says that *they specifically* are being controlled when they go to the fridge, then they are experiencing a delusion.

Those with OCD (see Chapter 6) often believe that they may be 'going mad' because of the thoughts they experience, but in OCD the person knows the thoughts are their own, even if they are unwelcome, while the person with delusions believes that these unwanted thoughts come from outside themselves or are inserted by external forces.

This group of symptoms (third-person hallucinations, thought alienation, and passivity) are known as Schneider's First Rank symptoms. This term was coined by German psychiatrist Kurt Schneider (1887–1967), who believed that these symptoms in particular were indicative of schizophrenia. It is now known that these can also be present in mania (see Chapter 7) or delirium (see Chapter 12), and so of themselves do not confirm the diagnosis of schizophrenia.

THE PRODROMAL PHASE

Schizophrenia frequently begins in the teenage years, and initially the symptoms may be vague, and include lack of motivation, social withdrawal from school, friends, family and hobbies. This may be attributed simply to teenage behaviour, and indeed sometimes this can be the case. This general withdrawal may be associated also with features such as hearing noises that are unusual or having a general mistrust of others. This is known as the prodromal phase. This is followed by the acute phase with *positive* symptoms. These are so-called because they are definite and include hallucinations and delusions. There are now services available for young people who may potentially be exhibiting the prodromal symptoms, and these early intervention services aim to intervene early to prevent progression of the condition. This period can last from months to years and this can delay the initiation of treatment for many years. A long prodrome is one of the factors associated with a poor outcome.

THE ACUTE PHASE AND POSITIVE SYMPTOMS

The delusions and hallucinations that are the core of schizophrenia are referred to as *positive* symptoms because these are the features that are obvious and bizarre. There will probably be definite auditory hallucinations, usually with the voice or voices speaking in the third person. There may be a feeling of being touched by something or of thought interference. A general sense that something strange is happening, known as *delusional mood*, is also reported. It is tempting to try to talk the person out of their beliefs and thoughts, but this may aggravate the situation and so caution is advised; it might be better to seek professional help directly.

The person may become extremely agitated and perplexed at this time, and if the symptoms are very distressing, admission to hospital may be required. This is a situation in which compulsory admission is required. The agitation experienced by the person may also be extremely distressing for the family, but when this happens a meeting with the consultant looking after the person may offer reassurance.

Some with schizophrenia develop depressive symptoms after the acute episode has passed. It used to be assumed that this was secondary to the knowledge of having a serious mental illness. Now, however, it is believed that the depressive features are part of the illness. They usually respond well to antidepressants, although the psychiatrist may choose to explore other possible environmental causes too.

THE LATER STAGE OF SCHIZOPHRENIA AND NEGATIVE SYMPTOMS

Some, but not all, of those suffering from a schizophrenic episode become withdrawn and lack motivation as the illness progresses or when relapse rates increase. In the past this was thought to be the result of institutionalisation, but now it is accepted as part of the illness process, particularly if there are repeated admissions due to relapses or under-treatment. The person also often displays problems with engaging in everyday affairs, and this can easily, but mistakenly, be attributed to laziness. The person may become socially withdrawn, and their mood may be 'flat' – in other words, it does not change when either positive or negative things happen to them. There is often lack of self-care too, and the person may feel detached from what is happening around them. Education, occupation and relationships become more difficult to sustain when these symptoms occur. Even with encouragement and rewards, these are features that are difficult to change. One particular medication, clozapine, has been found to help these negative symptoms. Changes to the part of the brain known as the lateral ventricles have been observed in those with these negative symptoms, and these changes, unfortunately, are difficult to change back. This is a very stressful situation for families and carers.

WHAT ABOUT SPLIT PERSONALITY? THIS HASN'T BEEN MENTIONED

Some refer to schizophrenia as a 'split personality'. This is one of the popular myths about schizophrenia. The word 'schizo' does mean split, but Eugen Bleuler, the man who coined the term 'schizophrenia' to describe the condition, was referring to the break between the person's thinking processes and emotions, not their personality. There is a controversial condition called dissociative identity disorder (see Chapter 10), previously referred to as multiple personality disorder, and this is likely to have contributed to this idea of a split in the personality.

CAN SCHIZOPHRENIA BY TREATED?

Schizophrenia can be treated. The mainstay of treatment is medication; psychotherapy also has a role, but this will only begin once the acute episode has settled and for very specific elements of the condition.

Medications

A first episode of psychosis has many causes (see p.134). When it is confirmed that the symptoms are those of schizophrenia, treatment is initially a course of antipsychotic medication for one to two years, and usually towards the longer end.

The older antipsychotic medications (called the first-generation group) began with the development of chlorpromazine in the 1950s (see Chapter 1). Other drugs in the first generation are listed in the first column below.

First-generation Antipsychotics	Second-generation Antipsychotics	Injectable (depot) preparations
• Chlorpromazine	• Aripiprazole (Abilify)	• Aripiprazole (Abilify)
• Fluphenazine	• Clozapine (Clozaril)	• Fluphenazine decanoate
• Clopenthixol	• Olanzapine (Zyprexa)	• Haloperidol decanoate
• Thioridazine	• Paliperidone (Invega)	• Paliperidone (Invega)
• Haloperidol	• Quetiapine (Seroquel)	• Risperidone (Risperdal Consta)
• Perphenazine	• Risperidone (Risperdal)	
• Amisulpiride	• Ziprasidone (Geodon)	

These are all associated with significant side effects, such as movement disorders, weight gain and drowsiness. None, with the exception of halo-peridol, are used very much now.

Second-generation antipsychotics were developed in the 1990s, and these have been shown to be as effective as the first-generation antipsychot-ics, but with different and usually less disabling side effects. These med-ications are listed in the second column above. A particular drug in this group is clozapine. This is used for those who do not show a response to the other drugs used in schizophrenia. It requires monitoring of blood levels of the drug to avoid toxicity and also monitoring of the person's blood pro-file, since it can reduce white cells, with potentially serious consequences. Second-generation antipsychotics may also cause weight gain and elevated blood sugars, which in turn can lead to diabetes. For this reason, weight checks and blood glucose levels are monitored every few months.

Preparations (referred to as depot injections) are available in long-acting injectable form and these are used for two groups. The preparations are listed in the third column in the box on p.141. There are some with schizoprhenia who do not want the bother of taking medication every day or perhaps be reminded that they have this illness. Getting an injection every three months allows them the freedom to forget about the illness and get on with their lives. These preparations are also used for those who experience frequent relapses, either because they do not take their tablets regularly or because they are unable to achieve steady levels in the blood for some biological reason. Administering the medication at set intervals (determined by the medication itself), from two-weekly to three-monthly, will help prevent relapse.

Psychotherapy

Psychological interventions are necessary to assist the patient in coming to terms with their illness, and at times to assist them in coping if they experience persistent hallucinations. They may also require skills in interacting with others, particularly if they have been ill for some considerable time and have lost the ability to socialise with ease.

They may also require vocational rehabilitation and, sometimes, if they have been unable to remain in their previous jobs or have been unable to obtain work in the open market, supported employment.

Family therapy is also required to provide support and education to the families, in particular to carers. They find it extremely stressful looking after a family member who may, as a result of the illness, be lacking in interest and motivation, may be having continuing psychotic symptoms, or may not be adhering to treatment. There is evidence of heightened rates of depressive and anxiety symptoms in that group.

Another reason for family therapy is that the family environment may trigger relapses in certain instances, a phenomenon known as *high expressed emotion* (high EE). This has been shown to cause relapses in situations where there is a tense relationship between the family and the patient. The elements of high EE are emotional over-involvement of members in the patient's life, criticism of the patient and hostility. In these circumstances the likelihood of relapse reduces significantly if the contact is reduced to fewer than 10 hours per week. High EE has to be distinguished from the now debunked theory that relationships within the family somehow *cause* schizophrenia. High EE triggers a *relapse* in an *already existing* illness, and this is an important distinction.

WHAT IS THE OUTCOME?

Both 10-year and 30-year follow-up studies have been conducted on those diagnosed with schizophrenia. They show that about 25% of those diagnosed make a complete recovery and have no further episodes, another 25% are improved to the point of being able to function independently, another 25% require significant support, a further 15% show little improvement with frequent hospitalisations, and 5–10%, unfortunately, die by suicide. However, these figures do not capture the broad spectrum of outcomes in individual patients (Jablensky, 2012). There is considerable individual variation in the outcome, and this is determined by a number of factors, listed below.

Factors affecting outcome

- How well the person functioned before becoming ill
- The time lapse from the occurrence of symptoms to beginning treatment (on average this is 6–7 years)
- Adherence to medication
- Avoiding non-prescribed and illegal drugs
- Having a supportive family
- Access to psychosocial interventions
- Insight into the early signs of relapse
- Absence of a family history of schizophrenia

In short, the numbers in the outcome studies mentioned above are not 'set in stone': if the right measures are taken, the odds of a good outcome can be increased.

ANTI-NMDA AUTOIMMUNE ENCEPHALITIS

This autoimmune reaction, causing inflammation of areas of the brain, resembles schizophrenia. This is a rare condition. The main presentation is with psychotic symptoms similar to those found in schizophrenia. There are few neurological symptoms despite the inflammation of these areas of the brain. The onset of psychiatric symptoms is commonly preceded by a viral illness with headaches and fever. Concentration and speech may be impaired, and this progresses to psychosis. Blood tests for inflammation may be only slightly elevated or even normal. A lumbar puncture will assist in making the diagnosis. Treatment is with steroids and antipsychotic medications. Recovery may take months to years. Some psychotic and mood symptoms may continue even after treatment (Pollack et al., 2019). This condition was captured in the movie *Brain on Fire* (2018), which tells the real story of a young woman who experienced this illness.

SCHIZOAFFECTIVE PSYCHOSIS

In this condition, bipolar disorder symptoms occur at the same time as the symptoms of schizophrenia. As with schizophrenia, antipsychotic medication is required along with antidepressants if the depressive pole of bipolar disorder is present. A mood stabiliser such as lithium is also required to control the mood swings. Pharmacological treatments are usually lifelong.

The causes of schizoaffective psychosis are under-researched but are likely to be similar to those of its component conditions. It occurs in about 0.3% of the population and is more common in women than men (this is the reverse of schizophrenia). In some respects it has a better outcome than schizophrenia since the negative symptoms mentioned above do not occur, but when depressive symptoms are present there is a heightened risk of suicide. Like any major mental illness, if under-treated, it too is associated with loneliness, isolation and problems with relationships.

DELUSIONAL DISORDER

This is a disorder that is not well known to the public, even though it is quite common. It occurs when there are delusions focusing on a particular person or occurrence. These conditions with single delusions are referred to as *monosymptomatic* delusions. Common delusions are of a persecutory nature, of infidelity, of love or of serious illness. Hallucinations and thought alienation do not occur. Because the symptoms are very circumscribed to one or two particular issues, the diagnosis can often be missed. Many people with this condition are able to work, maintain their self-care and have relationships. An exception to this is the person with delusions of their partner's infidelity (a variant known as the 'Othello' syndrome).

Case Vignette

A man aged 60 was brought to the emergency department by his family because his wife became fearful for her safety. He continued to work but insisted, for about two years, that she was being unfaithful. He was now threatening to do 'something' unless she desisted. When asked how he knew this, he responded that his wife was giving signs to her lover by causing the smoke from their chimney to twirl in a particular design. His wife attempted to reassure him that this was not true and showed him copies of her text messages to prove this. He refused to accept this reassurance. He had no other symptoms, such as hallucinations. His GP had previously referred him to the psychiatrist after his wife requested this, but he failed to attend.

Comment:
This man had delusions focusing on his wife's fidelity. She attempted to reassure him, and this is understandable but futile. He continued to work, and this is common when a person has a single, circumscribed delusion. Nobody would notice any problem with him. To those who are not the subject of the delusion, he seems perfectly well. Delusions with content of this nature are dangerous and the person may be at risk of being harmed. The person rarely accepts their illness and if prescribed medication rarely takes it. Sometimes it may be necessary to admit the person compulsorily. This man has a diagnosis of delusional disorder – his only symptom is a delusion of infidelity.

Note: This is not a real case but typical of the presentation of a person with delusional disorder.

Delusional disorder is sometimes associated with stalking. This behaviour occurs in the context of delusional beliefs that the stalker is loved by the other person (i.e. the stalkee). This is more common in females and the focus of the person's attention is often a celebrity or somebody who is otherwise of high status.

Delusions about health often focus on infestations. For example, the person will believe that there are unusual bugs in their skin that nobody can see. This condition is called *delusional parasitosis* and often leads to consultations with dermatologists. .

Sometimes a delusional person's concerns are so convincing that another person may come to believe that they are not in fact delusional. This other person is most often a family member, and it has even been known, albeit rarely, for this person to take on the delusions of the ill person. This shared delusion is known as *folie a deux*. Treatment involves separating the couple to allow the non-ill party to recover spontaneously. The ill person requires treatment.

Attempts at convincing the person that their beliefs are mistaken or that they are ill is impossible and may even reinforce the delusion, with sad consequences. Those with delusional disorder strongly resist taking antipsychotic medication. Psychological therapy may help provide support to the patient in the short term, but this usually ends when the person decides that the problem lies elsewhere and that they do not have any illness.

INDUCED PSYCHOSIS
See Chapter 11 for drug-induced psychosis, and Chapter 12 for delirium.

 WHAT YOU CAN DO FOR YOURSELF AND WHAT OTHERS CAN DO FOR YOU

- If you have a psychotic illness take your medication as prescribed.

- Avoid illegal drugs, e.g. cannabis or cocaine, because these can cause relapse.

- If you have a difficult relationship with your family try to reduce the amount of time you are with them.

- Keep in contact with your community mental health nurse.

- If you are a family member/carer, join a support organisation.

- Keep in touch with the community mental health nurse.

- Do not try to persuade your family member that their delusions are 'false' or that their voices 'are in the head'.

- If you are the focus of delusions do not try to prove their falsehood.

- If you are accused of infidelity because of delusions, consider leaving.

BIBLIOGRAPHY

Dean, Kimberly and Murray, Robin M. 'Environmental risk factors for psychosis'. *Dialogues in Clinical Neuroscoence.* 7,1. 69–80. 2005.

Pollack, Thomas A., Lennox, Belinda R., Muller, Sabine et al. 'Autoimmune psychosis: an international consensus on an approach to the diagnosis and management of psychosis of suspected autoimmune origin'. *Lancet.* 7,1. 93–108. 2020.

Jablensky, Assen. 'Course and outcome of schizophrenia and their prediction'. *New Oxford Textbook of Psychiatry* (2nd edition). Oxford: Oxford University Press. 2012.

USEFUL RESOURCES

Cockburn, Patrick and Cockburn, Henry. *Henry's Demons: A Father and Son's Journey out of Madness.* New York, NY: Scribner. 2011.

Shine – an organisation designed to support and empower all people with mental ill health. 01-5413715 or info@shine.ie

Mental Health Ireland – a charity that supports people with mental health problems and brings practical expression to national policy objectives. 01-2841166 or info@mentalhealthireland.ie

Dealing with Psychosis: A Toolkit for Moving Forward with Your Life. 2012. This online toolkit, funded by the British Columbia Ministry of Health is very user-friendly and covers relevant aspects of coping with schizophrenia.

Desperation, activism and light

I am a family member – the mother. My son was in hospital to have a rod removed from his femur which had fractured 18 months previously. The day came for him to be discharged and I went up to bring him home. I expected to find him dressed and packed and ready for me. But it wasn't like that. I entered the ward and saw him still in his pyjamas, aimlessly siting on a chair. He didn't greet me. I helped him to pack and dress, said Goodbye to the kind sister and we left.

He likes plants and gardens so I took us to a garden open to the public on the way home but he didn't seem interested. At home a friend came to visit and he ignored her. The next few days were increasingly difficult and I became afraid. He said I was a demon and many other disturbing things.

I contacted several psychiatrists, all of whom were either on holiday, about to go or had just returned. It was July. A medic myself, we didn't have a GP in those days. I phoned one I knew who kindly came out to the house. Our son stayed in his bedroom but eventually came down. While I was in the kitchen the GP miraculously persuaded our son to go to St John of God's Hospital – briefly, 'then I will come straight home'.

I took him up and he agreed to be admitted. It was to the locked ward and I was devastated. When I visited the next day he was crying desperately by the door.

I was shocked not to be given any information about him – for confidentiality reasons. I understood this but also felt the family to whom the patient would return when finally discharged would not know what to do and this would be unhelpful for both patient and family. With my medical background I felt in a better position than many of the relatives I spoke with in the hospital coffee room.

For several years I tried to address this – with psychiatrists, on the radio, with Schizophrenia Ireland (now Shine) with EUFAMI (a European-wide organisation that helps families living with severe mental illness) and other outlets.

Stigma is still a problem for those suffering from mental illness. It makes it difficult for the service user to apply for a job, and for family members to talk with other people. When our son first became ill he didn't want anyone to know and I found meeting other people challenging. They asked about our children and I felt awkward, changing the subject and avoiding specific answers. Our other children were away from home and neither they nor my husband wanted to be involved. I felt very alone. Schizophrenia Ireland were a wonderful support. When I collapsed in tears on their doorstep, they took me in, offered me counselling and put me in touch with a relatives' support group.

The medication for our son was not effective. His condition deteriorated and he made a serious suicide attempt. He swallowed 100 aspirins and was heading for the canal. Something made him turn back and go to St V Hospital. We were phoned with the news and went straight up to the hospital. He had been given charcoal and was drowsy. This proved to be a turning point. He was admitted to a medical ward with kidney and liver damage and at first was upset he had not succeeded in his attempt. I sat by his bed and on one occasion, while praying, I seemed to see a shining halo over his bed and believed he would come through it all.

When he was medically fit, he went to St JoG hospital for several months. He was diagnosed with bipolar disorder. He was put on medication, saw a consultant and psychologist, all of which were right for him. He was able to talk about the severe bullying he suffered in school and, talking with his siblings, we all remembered events in his teenage years when he was behaving in a disturbing way. With CBT he learned structures and tools for living each day. He still uses these tools.

He eventually went to RP rehab for two and a half years, during which time he worked on an art portfolio. From this he was accepted into three art colleges and chose to go to NCAD. He came out with a first.

He came home gradually to start a new life. He is diligent with his medication and has learned to plan and carry out projects. He is able to talk about his condition and experiences when appropriate and many people meeting him today would not realise his history.

I have worked on psychiatric wards, but through my own experiences as a family member have a greater understanding of the difficulties the patient and their family have to work through. I am immensely grateful for those who have been there for us with their skills to enable our son after many troubled years, now to live a normal life. Many thanks to God.

A mother fighting on her son's behalf

My son is now 51. He suffered a rare worm infestation when he was two. From then on he became very difficult to manage, very unpredictable, uncooperative, sometimes violent, yet could be good and loving. We sought help, diagnosed as having hyperactivity.

School was a nightmare, always in trouble. His education ended at 12 as he had to be expelled. I now firmly believe he actually had schizophrenia even then.

The years of trying to help and trying to get help for me, my son and the family are so painful to think of and I cry not just for myself, my other children, but mostly for N, who must have been in hell. Social life went almost out the window because as sure as shooting some disturbance would break out. Who would want to visit a house as mad as ours? I just wanted to love and cherish all five of my children, but so much had to be spent on N, the others lost out, and I felt such a failure.

Begging, begging for professional help, Neil been treated like an imbecile, me like a nuisance to be shooed away.

I found Schizophrenia Ireland, now known as SHINE, the first non-judgemental and support place around mental issues. Through its education and help I got a glimpse of how it must be for N. For me it shifted a gear to see N as a human being, not this big lump of inhumanity put on this earth to annoy and punish me.

I eventually had a breakdown myself and had to be hospitalised, such was the toll of fighting for N. I speak as if I am the only carer; my husband and other children have suffered, the shame of the mad son, brother, the disruptions of ordinary times, joyous times spoiled, the fear of him, the loss of him.

Our marriage lasted 50 years, it was good despite all the drama. He died five years ago.

None of my other children became Taoiseach, but at least they are not ashamed to be seen in the pub with me.

I am still in SHINE, and I made really good friends there. But what breaks my heart is new members telling how it is so hard to get help, to be listened to, patient confidentiality, when what we want to know is how to handle this frightening new situation we are in.

N is now with a team who are respectful of him and me and the ease of that is invaluable. He has his own supervised accommodation and manages really well. Thank God.

THE LIVED EXPERIENCE

Schizoaffective disorder and hope

After many years of suffering from mental health disorder I was in 2008 diagnosed as suffering from schizoaffective disorder. It manifests itself as periods of low mood and mania. It explains the many episodes of hospitalisation I underwent. I was relieved that at last I had a diagnosis for my illness. Since then I have been well with the medication of Epilim and olanzapine.

My first major breakdown occurred in 1996 when I attended a pro-life seminar with a Professor Philip Ney and Dr Marie Peeters from Canada. I was suffering from post-abortion trauma after undergoing an abortion in 1990. This seminar was for a week and involved group psychotherapy. We were encouraged to humanise our aborted child and go through a mourning process. Professor Ney considered abortion as a symbolic suicide. At the seminar we did visualisations. It was at this point I became unwell and began to hallucinate. I thought that Dr Marie Peeters was Jesus Christ. I thought that Christ had come back to earth and was here to heal women from suffering after their abortions. At this stage I didn't realise I was ill and I got more and more distressed when Dr Ney said I had to go to hospital. I didn't want to be separated from Marie Peeters as I believed she was Jesus. I became hysterical and could not be controlled. I ended up running away from the seminar and went missing for three days, staying in B&Bs.

After a number of days I phoned my parents and they found me and picked me up. I was still in a state of high anxiety and agitation, believing I had met Jesus Christ. My family finally convinced me to go to hospital and I was admitted to a mental health hospital. I was given Largactil, a major tranquiliser. Even though I was in a mental hospital I still believed I was a friend of Jesus. I was even more convinced when Dr Ney and Marie Peeters came to see me in hospital. I truly believed I was in the presence of God Almighty. I couldn't take my eyes off Marie and was transfixed.

Upon my discharge from hospital I was still in a state of ecstasy, waiting for when I would see Marie again. I wrote to her in Canada, believing still that she was Jesus, and was thrilled when she wrote back. My world came crashing down one day when I received a letter from her to say that she and Philip got married. I was devastated and couldn't believe what I was reading. I immediately went into a deep depression. I had nothing to cling to. I had in the meantime given up my job and lost a lot of friends. I was readmitted to hospital, this time with depression and low mood. I spent two weeks there without any improvement. My mood was so low that I contemplated suicide. They discharged me with some antidepressants. I lost the very thing I held dear to me – my Catholic faith. I couldn't believe God could treat me this way after all my prayers.

I was so lonely and depressed I retreated to my bedroom and effectively vegetated for a whole year. The antidepressants didn't work and I spent long hours watching TV and drinking to excess. I hated everyone and everything. My poor parents didn't know what to do with me. I longed for hours for the elation that my psychosis brought me. All my friends became estranged and didn't communicate with me as I was just an empty shell. All the hard work I had done on rehabilitation after my abortion came to nothing.

The following years, from 1996 to 2008, were periods of elation followed by the most terrible lows. I was hospitalised on numerous occasions, sometimes for depression and other times for elation. In 2008 I had the good fortune to meet a brilliant psychiatrist at a mental health hospital, and she finally diagnosed me with schizoid affective disorder. To have a name for my illness was a tremendous relief after all the wasted years of suffering. 2008 was the same year I joined the organisation called Shine. Shine is an organisation for people who experience mental health distress. We meet on a weekly basis and discuss any problems we have. It's a great outlet to have and I have made many great friends. We go on holidays together and have meals out on special occasions. So in 2020 life is good. I still have the normal ups and downs but nothing like the mood swings I experienced when undiagnosed. I am grateful to the support of the doctors and nurses and voluntary organisations who helped me recover from a serious illness. There is hope for everyone who suffers from mental health distress.

Is it asking too much to have more than half a life?

My brother had a bright future. Clever, funny, friendly, private school, honours degree; the world was his oyster. Yet even at the time of his graduation, something was happening that we couldn't define. A shift, a black cloud, a distancing. We started getting calls to collect him from Garda stations. He would wander up to strangers. 'Will you talk to me?' 'Why don't you like me?' The Gardaí turned him upside down looking for drugs, literally and physically. Our lives were going to turn upside down emotionally anyway.

There were no drugs. Something was happening internally. A malfunction that no one could see, no doctor could scan and no blood test would reveal. It was a long road to get the diagnosis of paranoid schizophrenia. After two years of unusual behaviour, he was locked bewildered in a cell and marched by the Gardaí into the psychiatric hospital and committed involuntarily. 'It's not a life sentence,' the psychiatrist told us. Oh how wrong he was.

My brother has never had a long-term job, never used his degree, never passed a driving test. People complain about a four-month lockdown; he has had a self-imposed lockdown for four years, broken only by six-monthly psychiatric appointments. He lives in fear. He sees people differently. Their expressions are as if through broken glass, sly and menacing. Their body language signals a personal threat. He is in danger and must hide, must stay in out of harm's way.

Multiple hospitalisations, longer each time, each one more futile than the rest. We can see the illness becoming more progressive, more ingrained, more part of him. Yet we still see flashes of him, on the good days, of what he once was, of his innate sensitivity, his compassion and his generosity. He feels persecuted, stigmatised, ostracised. Straight out of a locked room to home. 'We'll lock him in a cell and throw clozapine at him,' shouted a frustrated overworked psychiatrist to my elderly mother. 'He's tried clozapine several times,' she cries. 'It's the gold standard!' they reply in unison. How I wish the gold standard was compassion and understanding.

My mother is nearing 80, my father is dead. A brave face belies the dread she carries within her as state services let her deal with it alone with a sigh of relief. 'He causes trouble in the wards!' they complain. It's true, punch-ups happen. 'A conviction, let's bring him to court,' suggests the nurse. What happened to duty of care, we wondered. The rooms are double occupancy, if you're lucky, the bathrooms shared by many, the units tiny and crowded. Paranoid patients packed tooth by jowl is no recipe for wellness. Private healthcare does not cover a chronic disease like schizophrenia. It cannot cover the several months of hospitalisations. Don't get me wrong, we are indebted to the state when they have given him a bed rather than having him roam the streets. But is it really asking too much to have more than half a life? A handful of residential step-down, supportive, closely monitored facilities may be in existence. Never one that he has been able to access. We are very lucky. We can house him. Yet no one visits. The rare visit has been offered, but it is not with someone he knows.

Lack of continuity of nursing staff is an enduring problem. He needs a daily constant visit with a trained mental healthcare worker whom he knows and trusts. And true, often he will see it as spying, as antagonistic, as a ruse to get him locked up in that tiny ward again. I'm not saying the answers are easy, but neither should it be this difficult. My mother is afraid. She is afraid what will happen to him when she dies. She was the strongest person I knew, but this has broken her. She has no peace of mind. 2021 will mark 20 years since his diagnosis. Optimism, positivity, eroded to the bone.

Despite the buzzwords of mental health, schizophrenia still feels like a dirty word, full of blame and fear. Or the new euphemism of personality disorder. How far we have not come. And now I'm afraid for him, for her, and the cycle continues. We had no genetic history, we went through no wars, no violence. We were once you. We were once normal. We were once happy. If your child, your sister or your brother developed schizophrenia, how would you like them to be treated In Ireland in 2021? Would you want support, safety, understanding and compassion? Or would you want isolation, ignorance, fear, shame or suicide? I stopped him committing suicide. I promised him life would get better. That was 20 years ago. Should I have ever made that promise? It's one that I have failed to keep.

9

Suicidal Behaviour

'I felt suicidal' is a phrase we often hear. But what does it really mean when a person says they are suicidal? Did they really want to die? Are they likely to end their lives in the short term or even in the long term – or is it just an innocent way of indicating distress? It could mean one of several things, and one of the most important skills psychiatrists have to learn is how to interpret what is going on when people express themselves in this sort of way. If you or someone you know expresses themselves in the language of suicide, you need to discuss this with your/their GP sooner rather than later. It is a myth to assume that because somebody talks about suicide they will not do it.

Psychiatrists have a rich language for discussing suicidal language such as this. This chapter looks at some of the most important concepts and categories.

SUICIDAL THOUGHTS

Suicidal thoughts, suicidal plans, self-harm and suicide itself are all referred to as suicidal behaviour. And what any one person means when they say they are suicidal can vary with what they themselves believe it to mean. Note that self-harm counts as suicidal behaviour even if it is done without any suicidal thoughts or ideation. The reason for this terminological quirk is the close connection between self-harm and suicide. A list of the various suicidal behaviours and their definitions is provided on p.160.

Suicidal behaviours and their definitions

Suicidal ideation/ Thoughts	Thoughts of ending one's life
Passive death wish	A wish to die in one's sleep or accidentally, but without being actively involved in bringing it about
Active death wish	A positive desire to take one's life
Non-suicidal self-injury	An injury (e.g. an overdose or self-cutting) committed without the intention to die
Self-injury/suicide attempt	An injury committed with the intention to die
Suicide gesture	Self-injury without intent to die, but to give the appearance of a suicide attempt in order to communicate with others
Suicide	

Suicidal thoughts are common in the general population and even more so in those with mental health problems. Studies have examined this in several countries and have found that within any 12-month window, around 2% of the general population experience some form of suicidal behaviour. About 9% of people describe such thoughts as occurring at some point in their lives. The thoughts are most commonly fleeting and occur in the context of a personal crisis (e.g. break-up of a marriage, death of a loved one). They are generally not associated with any plan to harm oneself, and they disappear once the problem triggering them has lessened or as the person adapts to the situation. In situations such as this, the suicidal thoughts are best seen as a distress signal.

If someone starts forming a plan to end their life, however, it becomes appropriate to become more concerned. Hopelessness is also a symptom that may indicate despair, as is excessive guilt. A person who often stole sweets as a child now harbouring significant guilt about this, or a person who continues to have guilt about a previous matter for which they have made recompense would be examples. Frightening though talk of suicide is, most of those who have suicidal ideation have no plans to harm themselves: these are impulsive thoughts, usually in the context of a crisis. Nonetheless suicidal thoughts and actions must be taken seriously. In particular, when plans, hopelessness and/ or guilt are present, the person should be promptly evaluated by a mental health professional. This is most often in the emergency department of the local hospital; if a person is already under the mental health services, a member of that team should be notified. Thoughts at this level of seriousness are reported in less than 1% of the population.

SELF-HARM

Engaging in acts of self-harm is distressing for the person concerned as well as for their family. Self-harm can take many forms, such as cutting, overdosing, hanging, drowning and so on. The health service treats self-harm extremely seriously, and every person who presents at a hospital following self-harm undergoes a complete assessment of the psychological, social and biological factors that contributed to the act. This is a requirement of the National Clinical Programme for Self-Harm (NCPSH), which is a HSE/College of Psychiatrists of Ireland co-ordinated mental health programme aimed at reducing suicide. Since the biggest risk factor for suicide is whether a person has previously self-harmed, the NCPSH is an important initiative in tackling suicide in Ireland. It is part of the National Suicide Research Foundation (NSRF), which produces research papers and an annual report based on the data collected for the National Self-Harm Registry (www.nsrf.ie). This is one of the few such registries in the world, and is the most comprehensive. The national programme commenced in 2014 and includes every hospital in Ireland that has an emergency department. As such, Ireland is a global leader in this field.

The psychiatric evaluation happens whether the intention behind the act of self-harm was suicide or not. For mental health professionals it is the acts that are suicidal in their *intention* that are the most worrying. It is also the case, though, that an act that does not have suicide as its intent can nonetheless lead to death. For instance, a person who takes a large overdose of paracetamol in a fit of anger may not know that paracetamol is as dangerous to the liver as it is. Liver failure may develop rapidly and death is the consequence. Because of this, mental health professionals treat even this sort of self-harm very seriously.

We now have a lot of information on self-harm in Ireland thanks to the National Self-Harm Registry. From this we have learnt that over 11,000 people present to emergency departments every year on foot of an episode of self-harm. This figure is an underestimate, though, since about 12% who self-harm do not attend the emergency department, or attend but leave before they are registered. Of those presenting, about 15% leave before they are assessed psychiatrically. The figures available show that the rate of self-harm, irrespective of motivation, is 204 people out of every 100,000. Slightly more than half are women, and the rate is highest in females aged 15–19. One in every 139 girls or young women attends hospital following self-harm. Among men, the group aged 20–24 has the highest rate, amounting to one in 181 attending hospital after self-harm each year. Of the methods of self-harm, overdosing is the most common, followed by cutting, and almost one third of cases involve the concurrent use of alcohol. Self-harm is more common in urban than in rural areas.

As with suicidal thoughts, most self-harm occurs in the context of an interpersonal crisis and, increasingly, the use of illicit substances is in the background. Drugs like cocaine, cannabis, LSD and alcohol can induce low mood, and this may result in self-harm (see Chapter 11).

The diagnosis most commonly made in those who self-harm is emotionally unstable personality disorder. Information on the causes and treatment for this condition is provided in Chapter 10. This is not the only diagnosis, however: self-harm can occur in those with any psychiatric disorder, including adjustment disorder (see Chapter 4), depressive episode (see Chapter 7) and so on. About one third repeat the episode within one year, and 1% die by suicide in that time also.

THE PROCESS OF EVALUATING SELF-HARM IN THE EMERGENCY DEPARTMENT

When a person takes an overdose or self-harms in any way, even if it was an impulsive act or done without any suicidal ideation, they should attend the emergency department in their nearest hospital. This will allow the physical effects (which may take some time to fully manifest) to be treated, and it will also assist in determining if this action was driven by any psychiatric condition.

A person presenting to the emergency department will initially be seen by a member of the medical team, and any physical treatments required will be provided – including admission to a medical or surgical ward if necessary. The person will then be seen by a member of the psychiatric team, most commonly a highly trained nurse specialising in self-harm or a doctor working in psychiatry.

The evaluation will take place in a private room in the emergency department or, if the person has been admitted to a ward, they will be seen there. It will consist of an interview with the person who has self-harmed and, where possible, information will be sought from the next of kin and the person's GP. If the patient refuses to allow this, it is possible that the mental health professional doing the assessment could override the patient's wishes, depending on the degree of suicide intent that is present. Breaking confidentiality rarely arises in this situation, since most people after self-harm will allow a conversation with a relative/friend/GP as part of the assessment. Third-party information may help in providing a full picture of the episode (see Chapter 14) and of the level of intent associated with it.

In carrying out the assessment, several elements impinging on the person need to be examined. These are listed below.

Broad areas for evaluation in self-harm

- Suicide intent will determine if psychiatric admission is required to ensure the person's safety.
- Psychiatric diagnosis will determine what, if any, illness the person has, and what treatment is appropriate.
- Triggers will assist in identifying the areas for which specific help may be required, e.g. sudden loss of a job, acute grief.
- Risk factors will identify if these are amenable to alteration, e.g. housing problems, poor social supports.

Protective factors: These will be of assistance in determining whether the patient has resilience (e.g. having children, religious beliefs).

Questions about suicidal thoughts and plans are part of the evaluation and are not dangerous; neither do they increase the risk of suicidal behaviour. Talking about such things can be difficult, but it is essential to probe the person being assessed so that information about suicide plans, hopelessness, acts in anticipation of death and so on can be evaluated.

Based on the totality of the information available, a working diagnosis will be offered and a treatment plan developed. This can range from admission to hospital, to referral to a psychiatric service, to discharge back to the GP's care. Sometimes the clinical nurse specialist will arrange a follow-up appointment to ensure that the treatment plan is being followed through on.

In the course of the evaluation in the emergency department, most will express relief they are still alive. In a few cases, though, there is disappointment that their attempt was unsuccessful. In these circumstances, psychiatric admission is required; this is both for the person's own safety and to formulate a treatment plan. Those who are suicidal but refuse inpatient treatment can be certified under the Mental Health Act 2001 as they pose a risk to themselves. Those with personality disorder or substance misuse cannot be admitted to hospital compulsorily for these conditions per se; however, if they are suicidal, they can be admitted compulsorily for evaluation of their depressive symptoms. Compulsory admission involves the person's next of kin or some other person who will initiate the process. Details are provided in Chapter 14.

In those who are admitted to hospital with suicidal behaviour, there are two periods of heightened risk. The first is when medication first begins to work, within days to weeks. This is because of a notorious disconnect between the early improvement in the person's motivation and the longer period required for a reduction in suicidal thoughts. Close monitoring occurs at this time. A further period of risk occurs shortly after discharge from hospital when the person may be away from the sanctuary and safety of inpatient care and back in their own home. Families should be advised of this heightened risk prior to discharge, and close contact with the treating team and observation by the family is necessary.

SUICIDE IN IRELAND
The suicide rate in Ireland has been dropping for the past eight years, from a peak in 2011 of 12.1 people per 100,000 people in the population to 7.2 per 100,000 in 2018. The fluctuation in the rate has been in the

male population, with rates in women being relatively static. There have been changes in the age profile with rates being highest at present in the 45–54 age groups, for both men and women. The high rate in younger men discussed so much in the past decade has now reduced. Compared with other EU countries, Ireland has the seventh lowest suicide rate overall, though in men it has the 17th lowest rate.

Changes in suicide rate in Ireland 2011–18

Year	Number	Total rate per 100,000	Male rate per 100,000	Female rate Per 100,00
2011	554	12.1	20.2	4.2
2018	437*	9.0*	13.6*	4.5*

*correct as of 20.10.2020

Some of the reduction in suicide is probably attributable to the enhanced services provided by the National Clinical Programme for those presenting to the emergency departments described above. It may also be related to the somewhat reduced use of alcohol among young people, or it may be part of the natural swings that have been associated with suicide data in other countries.

When someone has died by suicide, there is an inquest to determine if the death was in fact by suicide. This will include an autopsy to determine the physical cause of death. A psychological autopsy, on the other hand, differs from this and is not routinely used in Ireland. A psychological autopsy is a detailed investigation that gathers information from multiple sources, such as GPs, psychiatrists, psychologists, employers, family and teachers, to examine the factors that might have impacted on the person prior to and around the time of death. These are usually conducted months, or even longer, after the death. In this way a picture is built up of the patient's psychiatric condition and their risk factors and triggers. The autopsies are carried out in the context of research studies rather than for inquests. There are some psychological autopsy studies in progress in Ireland at present (see, for instance, Arensman et al., 2019, who published the study proposal). A psychological autopsy study conducted in the North of Ireland (Foster, 1997) found that 90% had some type of psychiatric disorder but that this was less likely in those under 30.

Studies of this kind are important as they provide a picture of the risk factors for suicide and information on possible triggers. Studies to date come from other countries. These have shown that most of those who die by suicide have some type of psychiatric disorder – mood disorders are the most common, followed by substance misuse. However, there is geographic variation across countries in this respect. Suicide in all countries, except China, is higher in men than women, and the rates are highest in the older age groups, particularly those over 50. The high rate in young men in Ireland was a source of much comment in the past but this has now reduced and the age group most at risk are those aged 45–54.

The knowledge that mood disorders are the most common feature of those dying by suicide points to the importance of treatment for mood disorders. So this finding is not just some abstract statistic but something of direct relevance to real people.

The other risk factors are being male; being in the 45–54 age group; having a psychiatric illness; having had a prior episode of self-harm, particularly in the recent past; being divorced, widowed or separated; being unemployed; and being from socio-economic groups four and five. However, many people in the population possess some or even all of these features, yet do not die by suicide. Thus, we cannot predict suicide just by listing someone's risk factors.

CAN SUICIDE BE PREDICTED?

This leads to a common question that the public asks: why can we not predict those who are likely to die by suicide and intervene to save them? The difficulty here is basically that the risk factors that have been identified are not specific enough: as we have just seen they are also found, albeit less commonly, in those who do not end their lives. Studies have been conducted that applied the known risk factors to those being treated for psychiatric disorders, but this approach hugely over-predicted suicide – many more people were predicted to die by suicide than did in fact die in this way. The ratio was 1 to 99: i.e. for every 99 people predicted to die by suicide, only one did. (In statistical lingo, we say that the risk-factor approach has a huge *false-positive* rate.)

WHAT SHOULD ALERT YOU TO SUICIDE RISK?

If you know of somebody with a mental health problem who also has a prior record of having self-harmed, they are at risk of suicide. If they are not adhering to treatment, this will increase the risk. Feelings of hopelessness and social isolation are also risk factors.

There are a number of pitfalls that people fall into when trying to care for somebody who may be suicidal. These are:

- Accepting promises that they won't kill themselves even though they have suicidal thoughts.
- Being too fearful to ask about suicidal thoughts. It is understandable that a family member may not have the skill to do this but their GP should be asked to do this assessment.
- It might be assumed that the person's predicament makes suicidal thoughts understandable. But most people, even in desperate circumstances, do not resort to suicidal behaviour, so this person's view of their situation will be clouded by the gloom of low mood.
- Warnings may be ignored, e.g. making a will when in a depressed state, talking about suicide.

ANTIDEPRESSANTS AND SUICIDE

There was concern that antidepressants, particularly in the SSRI group, might cause suicide. Accordingly, a black-box warning was placed around all antidepressants. Is this concern justified?

The current medical position is that antidepressants, with the exception of fluoxetine (Prozac), are not licensed for use in those under the age of 18. For young adults from 18–25, there is an increased risk of suicidal thoughts and, possibly, attempts when on antidepressants, but the link between antidepressants and suicide is nevertheless very weak. In addition, the risk has been identified in those taking antidepressants for anxiety rather than for depression. This is due to the small numbers dying by suicide in this age group. In those over the age of 24 the risk of suicidal behaviour due to antidepressants has not been demonstrated, and they have a protective effect against suicide in the over 65s. So on the current evidence, it seems that at least for those over 25, antidepressants do *not* increase suicidality.

However the position regarding the current warning in the under-25 age group is still a matter for debate. Indeed, suicidal behaviour in this age group has increased in recent years, and this has been attributed to the decline in antidepressant prescription for those in this group who are suffering with severe depression. A revision of the black-box warning in this age group has been recommended (Fornaro et al., 2019). However, more research is needed.

What this means is that antidepressants seem not to cause suicide in those over the age of 18, even though the warning remains in place up to the age of 25. Indeed, in clinical practice antidepressants are used in this group despite the warnings – although their use has diminished. So if you are on antidepressants and aged 18–24, you should not stop them without considered discussion with a psychiatrist familiar with the scientific studies on this matter. Depressive illness is linked to suicide, and stopping the medication may itself lead to a relapse and suicidal behaviour.

SUICIDE BEREAVEMENT

The family of a loved one who dies by suicide experiences grief that differs from grief in other situations. Self-blame is common, as is anger. Within families, blame may attributed, and this may have serious consequences for the integrity of the family. Some feel shame that suicide has occurred and feel that people cannot sympathise with them, or may even avoid them, because of the circumstances of the loss. The subsequent inquest is particularly difficult and harrowing.

It is also worth stressing that there is no evidence for an increase in psychiatric illness in those bereaved by suicide compared to those bereaved otherwise. Nevertheless, many will require professional help to support them through the grief, and the evidence suggests that the support of others similarly bereaved is of most value to them.

WHAT YOU CAN DO FOR YOURSELF AND WHAT OTHERS CAN DO FOR YOU

If you're feeling suicidal
- Tell somebody if you have impulses or thoughts of harming yourself.
- Do believe that even in very difficult situations things can improve.
- Do not drink alcohol or use illegal drugs to help you to feel better.
- Visit your doctor if you have thoughts of harming yourself.

If you're worried that someone you know may be suicidal
- If your loved one has thoughts of suicide do not ignore this.
- If they have thoughts of suicide, try to persuade them to attend their doctor.
- If they tell you about their suicidal thoughts do not get angry or refuse to talk about it.
- If they tell you about suicidal thoughts do not falsely reassure them – they may feel you don't appreciate the depth of their sadness.

BIBLIOGRAPHY

Arensman, E., Larkin, C., McCarthy, J. et al. 'Psychosocial, psychiatric and work-related risk factors associated with suicide in Ireland: optimised methodological approach of a case-control psychological autopsy study'. *BMC Psychiatry.* 19,1. 275. 2019.

Fornaro, M., Annalisa, A,. Valchera, A. 'The FDA "Black-Box" warning on antidepressant suicide risk in young adults:more harm than benefit'. *Frontiers in Mental Health.* DOI. 3 May 2019.

Foster, T., Gillespie, K., McLelland, R. et al. 'Risk factors for suicide independent of DSM-111 axis 1 diagnosis. Case-control psychological autopsy study in Northern Ireland'. *British Journal of Psychiatry.* 175. 1175–791. 1997.

National Suicide Research Foundation (www.nsrf.ie)

USEFUL RESOURCES

Schreiber, Jennifer J. and Culpepper, Larry. 'Suicidal ideation and behaviour in adults'. UpToDate website. October 2020.

Arensman, Ella, McAuliffe, Carmel, Corcoran, Paul et al. *First Report of the Suicide Support and Information System.* Cork: National Suicide Research Foundation. 2012 (available online).

Wertheimer, A. *A Special Scar: the experience of people bereaved by suicide.* London: Routledge. 2001.

Pieta House Head Office 01-4585490; and for those bereaved by suicide 1800-247247 or www.pieta.ie/

Samaritans Ireland 01-6710071; or your local number or www.samaritans.org

Repeated self-harm

My first interaction with mental health came when I was 15 years of age. In secondary school, my best friend was a 'Goth' and I was a 'nerd'. She was carving images into her arm and I wanted to look cool so I copied her with a compass. When I was bullied for different things throughout my secondary school years I used that compass again and again to hurt myself and it felt good. It relieved the shitty feelings I felt when I didn't stand up for myself. I did get some counselling in school but only after I was made to tell a teacher about my sexual orientation. The counselling lasted exactly five sessions because the school could not afford the counsellor. I didn't think much of the counsellor. I felt I wasn't doing much harm to anyone, let alone myself.

My next interaction with mental health and the first encounter with the mental health services was my second job in a car garage, it was my first proper job after completing a PLC course. I felt great, I was working as a receptionist and an accounts assistant. I was 21 years of age when I left the job. This job and the manager left me hating myself so much that more often than not I prayed I would be hit by a car on the way to work, or I would die in my sleep on a Sunday night so I didn't have to turn in on a Monday morning. I left telling them I had another job opportunity. I didn't really. I had to leave because I was self-harming all the time and my family were seriously worried for my safety. I contacted my doctor and spoke with him. He put me on an antidepressant while I waited to access the mental health services in Portlaoise. I didn't have to wait long. My mind gets a bit blurry around this period. I think I may have spent a few days or a small period of time in the local psychiatric department but I was given counselling almost immediately. I spent a time with the psychologist who, after an assessment and a couple of sessions, gave me a diagnosis of borderline personality disorder with generalised anxiety disorder.

FEARS, PHOBIAS AND FANTASIES

From that first time right up to now as I am typing this I have been with the mental health services in P and an inpatient at times in the department of psychiatry there. I am no longer ashamed to say I have mental health issues and I self-harm. Yes, I still self-harm, and I am now 32 years of age. It's something I just can't give up and no one forces me to try and stop cold turkey. Self-harm has been there for me when family and friends gave up on me, it's been there for me when I was raped and sexually violated and I was sure no one wanted me around.

I have good and solid consistent help from the MDT in the T. Mental Health Centre and my psychiatrist Dr. D. They have helped me so much, I cannot thank them enough, especially of late, as I have had psychosis and it has been such a scary time. Every one of them has reached out to help me in any possible way they could, and at times when I have been vexed and given out they didn't turn their backs on me. They came back time and time again to ensure that I get the best help and treatment that is available to me.

– AO'B

– 172 –

10

Disorders of personality and behaviour

The idea of personality being disordered is very difficult for most people to grasp. After all, are we not all, in some way imperfect? Surely we *all* have difficulties at times with how we relate to others, and thus difficulties with our personality? Is the notion of 'personality disorder' not too judgemental? Indeed, because of all this, and because the diagnosis is so stigmatising, it is a condition that psychiatrists are reluctant to diagnose (Paris, 2007). In the past it was viewed as an innate weakness and regarded as untreatable. Such therapeutic nihilism deterred research that might identify therapies. It also resulted in a situation where some who had personality disorder co-occurring with another psychiatric disorder, e.g. generalised anxiety, were not being offered treatment for their anxiety. These attitudes have changed somewhat in the last decade, although there is still a residual reluctance to diagnose it.

A further concern is that sometimes schizophrenia is thought to be a type of personality disorder, popularly referred to as 'split personality'. This is incorrect. Schizophrenia is not a type of personality disorder and the confusion arose because the term 'splitting' was originally used to describe a splitting from reality (see Chapter 8) and, more recently, in neuroscience, to depict disorganisation in the brain circuits transmitting information.

However, personality disorder (PD), as defined by the WHO, the APA and by psychiatrists and psychologists working in the area, is much more than just the normal foibles of personality that we all possess. It refers to *enduring aspects* of one's psychological make-up that result in *continuing dysfunction* in day-to-day living. It manifests itself from the teenage years onwards. It impacts on our family, our workmates and our acquaintances. For example, an individual with personality disorder may continually alienate others, may be dependent on people throughout their lives for decision-making, or may be frequently aggressive for very minor reasons. It is accepted that we all, at times, undergo difficulties in our relationships, but personality disorder is distinct by being not just *occasional*, but consisting in *persistent* problems in how we relate to others. These are not related to the transient difficulties that occur when somebody is in the throes of a mental illness; rather, they are ingrained in the person's make-up.

Within mental health legislation personality disorder is dealt with differently from other disorders. There are also differences between countries in the legislation dealing with compulsory admission. For instance, in Ireland, an individual diagnosed with a personality disorder cannot be detained compulsorily just for that reason. So, if a person is aggressive and constantly attacking others because of a personality disorder, but does not have any other diagnosis (such as schizophrenia), they cannot be detained. This is different in England and Wales, where people *can* be detained for such behaviour. There are similar differences between countries throughout Europe.

The psychiatric textbooks and scientific literature have identified various types of personality disorder; these are listed on p.177. One of the problems with the current taxonomy is that for the most part, none of these have been proven to be independent of the others; indeed, many co-occur and overlap. So an individual who is very aggressive and hostile may also be persistently anxious, worrying, withdrawn and aloof.

HOW DO I KNOW IF I HAVE A PERSONALITY DISORDER?

The evaluation of personality is not based on one interview with an individual but on information garnered over time, mainly from other people, but of course also from the person themselves. Sometimes people are unaware of their own failings, and it is probably correct to say that this applies to most of us. The optimum way to assess personality is with an interview with the individual themselves, discussing how they react in different circumstances and how they believe themselves to be when they are well. This interview should be followed by interviews with others who have known the person throughout their lives and who can attest to their long-standing behaviours and traits. A person's personality is essentially determined by long-standing traits and enduring ways of relating to themselves, to close family and to others in their vicinity.

WHAT CAUSES PERSONALITY DISORDER?

Not enough is known about PD to be definitive about causes. There may be a genetic element, particularly in relation to antisocial/psychopathic PD. For other subtypes, the person may have experienced childhood traumas such as separation from parents – separation from one's mother seems to be particularly relevant. Others may have witnessed violence in the family as young children. This may influence how they form relationships with others, which, in turn, may lead them to becoming overly dependent on others. For other subtypes again, the cause may have been major childhood trauma such as sexual or physical abuse or neglect. Severe bullying at school may also be causal. For some, there seems to be a combination of both environment and genetic factors at play.

As people grow up personality mellows, and some traits, such as impulsiveness and aggression, reduce as the brain matures. On the other hand, some of the negative features such as rigidity, suspiciousness and anxiousness may continue or even worsen with age.

HOW IS PERSONALITY DISORDER DIAGNOSED?

Very few people go to their doctor, psychiatrist or therapist saying, 'I think I have a personality disorder'. This is because people know very little about PD. Many people have never heard of it, and those who have believe it to be a diagnosis to be concerned about. For this reason, it should be diagnosed with great caution. The diagnosis is almost always made from the history that the person gives and the history is usually a long-standing one of difficulties in relationships with others, be they people to whom the person is close, such as partners, siblings and spouses, or those more remote, such as employers, employees or even neighbours.

They may be very rigid and inflexible. They may be very anxious and dependent, and sometimes withdrawn and uninterested. Others may be very melodramatic, seeking constant attention, and others may be cruel and harsh. It is important that this evaluation comes not just from people who are close to the individual, such as partners and children, since such relationships can often be fraught in themselves, but from people who are less intimately connected to the person but who know them through work or as neighbours. This clinical practice approach may be assisted by other evaluations.

There are some therapists who assess personality using pencil and paper tests. Some of these tools are available online. The Minnesota's Multiphase of Personality Inventory (MMPI) (Hathaway and McKinley, 1940) test is one of the best known of these. Caution is required in using pencil and paper tests; they have a tendency, particularly when the individual completes them themselves, to lead to over-diagnosis of PD. The diagnosis of PD should ideally be made on the basis of the person themselves, but more especially those who know the person well, either through familial ties or through close relationships in other contexts, providing a history to a psychiatrist. This can be done along with a diagnostic and pencil and paper test. Note that even those tests that can be filled out online need to be interpreted with great caution.

WHAT TYPES OF PERSONALITY DISORDER OCCUR?

Some of the words that describe particular personality disorders are also used in everyday language. Terms like psychopathic, paranoid, obsessive and schizoid are common in our everyday language. However, when these are used in a psychiatric context they have a very different and specific meaning that differs from their meaning in everyday use.

Traditionally a number of personality disorder types have been described. Some have these have entered everyday language, such as passive-aggressive and narcissistic personality disorder. Another, formerly called multiple personality disorder, but now called dissociative identity disorder (DID), is described in Chapter 13.

Personality disorder categories familiar to the public

CATEGORY	FEATURES
Paranoid	Guarded, defensive, mistrustful, suspicious, difficult to work and be with
Schizoid	Withdrawn, emotionally cold and detached, loner
Antisocial	Odd, eccentric, strange beliefs, interested in occult, few friends
Emotionally unstable PD (EUPD), also called borderline PD (BPD)	Impulsive, quick-tempered, thoughtless, selfish, emotionally unstable, rapid shifts between idealising and hating, feelings of emptiness and abandonment
Histrionic	Dramatic, seductive, attention-seeking, self-absorbed, suggestible
Narcissistic	Arrogant, grandiose, sense of entitlement, sense of own superiority
Avoidant	Self-conscious, shy, easily embarrassed, low self-worth, socially tense
Dependent	Submissive, difficulty with decisions, reassurance-seeking, fragile
Obsessional (anankastic)	Rigid, formal, hidebound by rules and regulations, punctilious, organised
*Passive-aggressive	Resists suggestions, deliberately thwarts, undermines others' suggestions, shows aggression indirectly
*Self-defeating	Defeats own goals, forms friendships with condemning partners

*These conditions are no longer included in the US classification system (DSM-5).

These labels derive from the terms originally used to describe the dominant traits in individuals with PD. Psychiatrists first describing PD may have been over-zealous in creating a rich taxonomy of types of PD. Studies in recent years have shown that some of these overlap with others, and traits of one category are also found in another, so they cannot be regarded as existing in their own right. They have been withdrawn from use. From 2022 onwards the categories listed on p.177 will not be in use in Ireland or in the rest of Europe This is because ICD is the primary diagnostic manual throughout the world; the US DSM, however, will continue to use them.

What ICD-11 is proposing is that there will be three levels of severity – mild, moderate, severe – with six trait domains that include borderline, dissocial, obsessional and so on. It is likely to be cumbersome and not user friendly. Also, despite the shortcomings of the categories listed on p.177 and familiar to many, patients, their families and psychiatrists like a specific label and may not welcome this radical change.

HOW COMMON IS PERSONALITY DISORDER?
PD is present in about 13% of the general population (Volkert et al., 2018), with the obsessional and antisocial types the most common. In clinical settings such as psychiatric outpatients, PD is diagnosed in about 50% of those attending (Keown et al., 2002), although this is likely to co-occur with another psychiatric condition, such as depressive illness.

The obsessional group do not often present to psychiatrists since they are usually hardworking and diligent. It is those close to them who experience the greatest problems, due to their rigid behaviours and attitudes. Likewise, the antisocial group seldom seek help, due to lack of insight and a tendency to deny responsibility for their actions, and instead blame others.

The two categories that place the greatest demands on their families, on society and on mental health services by their behaviour are EUPD and antisocial PD. These will be described in further detail.

Emotionally unstable personality disorder
Those with EUPD represent about 1.9% of the general population (Volkert et al., 2018) but are the group who most often present to the emergency departments with self-harm. Their low and fluctuating moods, along with repeated episodes of self-harm, cause distress to themselves and others, and this is often what leads to their seeking help. They are divided into two broad categories: the *borderline* and the *impulsive* types. It was thought that the borderline group lay somewhere between the

neuroses (anxiety, panic disorder etc.) and the psychoses (schizophrenia and other conditions in which there is a loss of contact with reality causing delusions and hallucinations), but this way of seeing the condition no longer exists. Nowadays, borderline and EUPD are used interchangeably. The behaviour associated with EUPD invariably begins during the teenage years with self-cutting and fluctuating moods. It appears to be much more common in females than males in hospital settings, but this may be because women are more likely to *present* to hospital after an episode of self-harm, rather than simply because they are more likely to self-harm. This group often self-harms repeatedly, usually for the relief of tension rather than with any intent to end their life. This is referred to as *non-suicidal self-injury* (see Chapter 9), and may occur in response to stressful events and with varying levels of suicide intent. Anger is often to the fore, typically originating in their past trauma.

People with EUPD also frequently engage in substance misuse; this is for the same reason, as well as to suppress the painful childhood memories with which EUPD sufferers are often burdened. Because of their use of illicit drugs sufferers also frequently get into debt, often have trouble with the law, and may be impulsive financially, sexually and in their eating patterns (they will often engage in binge eating). The combination of a psychiatric disorder such as EUPD with substance misuse is termed *dual diagnosis* and can be difficult to treat. Some UK services engage specialists in dual diagnosis to help this complex group.

The suicide rate is higher than in the general population because of their impulsivity. About 10% of those with EUPD die by suicide, usually due to their repeated episodes of self-harm. Even those who do not die by suicide often have longstanding suicidal ideation, although the intensity varies. This is very distressing and worrying for family members. Managing longstanding and varying suicidal thought is clinically challenging, and families beg for admission to hospital. These requests are often denied because admission is not actually helpful except when the person is actively suicidal at the time. Sometimes brief psychotic episodes, called micro-psychoses, may occur. These often last no more than a few minutes but may last up to an hour, and they are triggered by stress. Medication is usually not required as they resolve spontaneously. The National Institute of Health and Care Excellence has issued guidance on the treatment of EUPD (CG,78).

Case Vignette

Joan, aged 23, was referred to the emergency department because she had taken an overdose. She had been in third-level education but dropped out because she had lost most of her friends and she felt lonely. She was also unsure if her course was suited to her – she was studying childcare. Now, 18 months later, she was unemployed and living in a house with other girls, with whom she did not get on. She kept to herself and spent her days watching TV, eating junk food, and drinking. She had gained a lot of weight. She would have between one and two bottles of wine over the course of an evening once or twice each week. On these occasions she felt lonely and empty and would cut herself. This relieved her distress.

She reported being low in mood since her teenage years, but this would fluctuate, and she had periods of a few days when she was happy and others when she was sad. She began cutting occasionally as a teenager. Her parents saw her do it once when she was 14 and tried to persuade her to attend the GP but she absolutely refused and promised not to do it again. Despite this, she continued to cut herself, but started focusing on her abdomen and thighs so as to conceal it from her parents.

She had done well at school until the age of about 10 when a caretaker had sexually abused her. This happened on a few occasions thereafter until he retired from his position. She never told anybody about this. She still had dreams about it and hated looking at her body. She was glad she had now gained weight as she believed she was less likely to be abused if she was unattractive. She had been in a few relationships with boys as a teenager, but these tended to be short-lived as she could not trust them, especially when sexual activity was suggested. She said they found her to be 'heavy going'.

Comment:
This presentation is very common. Symptoms will be present for several years before presentation and the person will usually seek help after an overdose, cutting or some other form of self-harm. Usually the episodes are not planned in any detail and in themselves have low intent. There is the inevitable risk of death, even if not explicitly planned, when an overdose goes wrong. The history of sexual abuse is very common, but the trauma may also be physical abuse, neglect

or severe bullying. Reluctance to disclose what has happened is also a problem, and this compounds the negative reaction that follows. There is good evidence that disclosing abuse or bullying – and being believed – helps prevent the negative consequences on mood, relationships and personality. The problems with interpersonal relationships described in this vignette are typical of EUPD also.

The treatment of choice is psychological, and dialectical behaviour therapy (DBT), a form of meditation and CBT combined, has the best evidence. If this is not available, then CBT and mindfulness are helpful in controlling symptoms. Despite the low mood described in this example, Joan also mentions that it fluctuates rapidly and that she has both good and bad periods. Medication does not help with these mercurial mood shifts, which differ from the more sustained changes seen in bipolar disorder.

Note: This is not a real case, but it describes a typical scenario.

Antisocial personality disorder

This is the term that is used for those who show disregard for the norms of social behaviour, who, because they exploit others, have difficulty maintaining relationships, and blame others for their life's problems. They cause great problems for society because of their explosive outbursts, their attitude to social norms and their impulsivity, which frequently comes to psychiatric attention and also brings them into conflict with the law.

They also frequently break the law and tend to be angry and aggressive, and may hit out for minor reasons. At their most severe, there is lack of guilt for the suffering they cause, and they are unable to learn from their mistakes. Psychopathy is the term used to describe those at the most severe end of this spectrum of behaviour: those who get pleasure from hurting others and who engage in the most severe and perverse levels of violence. Antisocial PD is more common in males than females, although whether this is a true finding or simply due to gender bias is unclear.

Those with antisocial PD normally have a history of conduct disorder in childhood that includes truancy, drug abuse from a young age and being aggressive and disruptive. It often develops in the child against a background of difficult family circumstances, with harsh unloving parents, alcohol misuse and violence. Imprisonment, substance misuse, self-harm and homelessness are common. The condition tends to lessen with time.

CAN PERSONALITY DISORDER BE TREATED?

Unfortunately for those afflicted with PD, demonstrable benefit from treatment is, for the most part, limited. Treating PD requires hard work and commitment from the individual concerned. Many do not wish to have therapy because they lack the insight to accept that their personality impinges negatively on others. Some blame the person or people with whom they have difficulties instead of acknowledging their own contribution to the difficulties. Others do not have the willingness to continue to attend. Generic interventions such as CBT may assist, but there are few therapies developed for most of the specific categories of PD.

EUPD and antisocial PD are the two categories for which treatments are most often suggested. Some studies have identified therapeutic approaches that may be beneficial in treating these types of PD. However, these treatments are time-consuming and not readily or universally available in Ireland.

EUPD has received a lot of attention and some people with EUPD benefit from a special treatment termed *dialectical behaviour therapy*, a combination of mindfulness and CBT. Mindfulness on its own is also used, as is mentalisation, a form of therapy that assists the person in understanding how they may unknowingly be exploiting others and how their behaviour affects not just themselves, but also those with whom they have relationships. Those with EUPD have a reduced capacity to mentalise. Even without treatment the mood instability tends to improve with increasing age.

The basics of DBT

INDIVIDUAL THERAPY	GROUP THERAPY	THERAPIST CONSULTATION	COACHING ON DEMAND
Therapists target self-injury and self-sabotaging behaviours	Focuses on distress tolerance and interpersonal effectiveness	Therapists meet to review their work and get feedback	Short, over-the-phone, coaching sesions that help overcome daily challenges

Medication is of little assistance in treatment of EUPD except when low mood is persistent, and even then it may not be effective. Mood stabilisers do not help either.

Treatment of antisocial PD is difficult and a person so diagnosed will often only agree to this when ordered by a court. CBT and anger management are sometimes used for this group, as are therapeutic communities. The National Institute for Health and Care Excellence in the UK has published guidelines on the management of antisocial personality disorder (CG,77) (2013). Medication such as lithium or carbamazepine may reduce aggression, but there is no evidence that medication can cure antisocial PD. Some people mellow with age, and with this maturation anger and impulsivity become less problematic.

STALKING

Stalking will be considered in this chapter, because although there are many mental health reasons for this behaviour, PD is probably the most common.

Stalking is defined as *repeated attempts by an individual to make contact or approach another person in a manner which causes distress, and which any reasonable person would realise was unwelcome and upsetting.* In its most severe form, it can be driven by delusions occurring in the context of psychosis. The contact may be physical, but it can also be in the form of emails, letters or telephone calls, or effected through social media.

In the UK around 12% of the population (Budd, 2000) report being stalked at some time in their lives, but certain professions are more at risk than others. Psychiatrists, police officers and social workers are particularly vulnerable because of the work they do with disturbed people. Celebrities are also at risk.

Stalking most commonly arises in the context of an intimate relationship that is in trouble or broken. The stalker knowingly follows the victim to check on their actions if they are jealous of them, or tries to communicate with the individual if they have been rejected or feel they have been treated unjustly. Celebrities are often stalked because of 'unrequited love'.

The impact on the victim can be significant, and when it continues for a long time can result in major psychological and social difficulties. For example, some people will not go out of their home for fear of being stalked. Others will change their telephone number or not go to work lest they be followed. Some feel forced out of their home. There are realistic safety issues at stake too, since a significant number of those stalked are also threatened. Anxiety symptoms, insomnia, impaired concentration and hyper-vigilance regarding the person's presence are among the symptoms that are found in victims of stalking.

In most instances, stalking stops after a few days, but those who have been stalked for more than around two weeks are strongly advised to contact the Gardaí. On no account should the individual make contact or communicate with the stalker. When stalking is associated with pathological jealousy it can be dangerous, and the full force of the law should be brought to bear on the individual who engages in this behaviour. That person may also be in need of psychiatric treatment. Ultimately, whether this is a psychiatric or a criminal issue needs to be established by the psychiatrist.

The victim may also need medication for symptomatic treatment of insomnia and anxiety, and may additionally need support in managing whatever actions they take to end the stalking.

ADULT ATTENTION DEFICIT HYPERACTIVITY DISORDER

Adult Attention Deficit Hyperactivity Disorder (adult ADHD) is an uncommon condition. Also called hyperkinetic syndrome, regular ADHD (i.e. not adult ADHD) is most commonly found in children, and by the age of 18 it has usually lessened significantly. It was once believed that after this age threshold it did not exist, but psychiatrists and patients now know that it can continue into adult life in a small proportion of people.

ADHD is one of the most controversial diagnoses in children because of its history of being over-diagnosed and over-prescribed. Since the drugs mainly used to treat the condition in children are psychoactive amphetamine-like substances, this further increases the general anxiety about the condition. Some believe that the 'wave' of ADHD – up to 30% of boys in some centres in the US have been diagnosed with it – is nothing more than misdiagnosed conduct disorder. This wariness of over-diagnosis has had a knock-on effect on discussion about adult ADHD.

Adult ADHD seldom presents for the first time in adulthood, except on the rare occasions that the symptoms, present since childhood, were not attended to, and present when the young person, usually a male, is having problems with concentration and attention for no apparent reason. If you had these features in childhood, even if you were not diagnosed, then you may have adult ADHD if these features have continued. The areas in which problems are noticed are listed below.

Problem areas in ADHD

- Organisation, e.g. planning and prioritising tasks
- Focus, e.g. maintaining focus and reducing distraction
- Memory, e.g. forgetting items such as clothes, forgetting recent events
- Persistence, e.g. maintaining effort, not exhibiting restlessness
- Impulsivity, e.g. regulating decision-making

In order to make the diagnosis it is important to attend a psychiatrist and/or clinical psychologist with experience in making the diagnosis. A number of pencil and paper tests will be carried out by the psychologist, while the psychiatrist will delve into the person's history in some detail and will also speak to somebody who has known the person for many years. Some of the features of ADHD are present in those with depressive illness, in those who are struggling academically because they dislike their course, and in those abusing substances. So if you think you may have adult ADHD it is important that these conditions are first ruled out when the diagnosis is being considered.

TREATMENT

Medications such as dexamphetamine or methylphenidate are used frequently for this condition. Non-stimulant medications like atomoxetine are also used, as is bupropion, an antidepressant. These will typically be used in those for whom psychostimulants cannot be prescribed because of prior drug abuse.

Life coaching and counselling are also advisable in helping people with prioritising work, helping self-esteem and assisting in coping with past failures.

WHAT YOU CAN DO FOR YOURSELF AND WHAT OTHERS CAN DO FOR YOU

Personality disorder
- Listen when others tell you that you may need therapy for your behaviour.
- If you constantly fall out with people, this may indicate that you need professional help.
- Read about others who have problems similar to yours.
- Discuss your problems with a mental health professional.

Stalking
- If you are the victim of stalking do NOT try to reason with the stalker.
- If it persists, report it to the Gardaí.

ADHD in adults
- Use reminders, such as notebooks.
- Have a structure to your day and keep a timetable.
- Declutter regularly.
- Put electronic tags on important items like wallets, keys etc.

BIBLIOGRAPHY

Budd, Tracey, Mattinson, Joanna, Myhill, Andy. *The extent and nature of stalking: findings from the 1998 British Crime Survey*. London: Home Office Research, Development and Statistics Directorate. (2000).

Hathaway, S. R. and McKinley, J. C. . 'A multiphasic personality schedule (Minnesota): I. Construction of the schedule'. *Journal of Psychology*, 10, (1940) 249–54.

Keown, P., Holloway, F,. Kuipers, E. 'The prevalence of personality disorders, psychotic disorders and affective disorders amongst the patients seen by a community mental health team in London'. *Social Psychiatry and Psychiatric Epidemiology*. 2002; 37: 225–9.

National Institute for Health and Care Excellence. 'Antisocial personality disorder: prevention and management'. [CG, 77] March 2013.

National Institute for Health and Care Excellence. 'Borderline personality disorder: recognition and management'. [CG, 78] January 2009 (rechecked 2018, no change).

Paris, J. 'Why Psychiatrists are Reluctant to Diagnose Borderline Personality Disorder'. *Psychiatry* 4,1. 35–9.

Volkert, J., Gablonski, T. C. and Rabung, S. 'Prevalence of personality disorders in the general adult population in Western countries: systematic review and meta-analysis'. *British Journal of Psychiatry*. 213,6. 709–15. 2018.

USEFUL RESOURCES

ADHD Ireland email: info@adhdireland.ie

https://www.rcpsych.ac.uk/mental-health/problems-disorders/adhd-in-adults This leaflet on the Royal College of Psychiatrists Website lists very useful self-help books.

www.bpdworld.org – a website with information on EUPD

Youtube, 'A live Dialectical Behaviour Therapy Session Explained' (5 June 2020) https://www.youtube.com/watch?v=Q9Zkfekeggs

Barkley, R. A., with Benton, C. M. *Taking Charge of Adult ADHD*. New York, NY: Guilford Press. 2010.

Gaynor, Keith. 'Embracing Borderline Personality Disorder' (an online talk on EUPD). 'An interview with a sociopath'. YouTube .10 February 2020.

Gentry, W. D. *Anger Management for Dummies*. For Dummies. 2006.

Lancer, D. 'Loving Someone with Borderline Personality Disorder'. Psych Central. 8 October 2018.

National Institute for Health and Care Excellence. 'Antisocial personality disorder: prevention and management'. [CG, 77] March 2013.

Partakovsky, Margarita. 'How to Help a Loved One with Borderline Personality disorder Part 1'. Psych Central. 8 October 2018.

THE LIVED EXPERIENCE

EUPD – relief at getting a diagnosis

———

Shame. Guilt. Empty. Alone. Worry. Fear.

These are just a few of the words I use to describe the thoughts that come into my head every hour of every day.

Crazy. Annoying. Burden. Stupid. Anxious. Complicated.

These are just a few of the words I use to describe myself when I am feeling low.

All of these words combined is what I currently feel as I am writing this. This is mainly because for the first time in my life, not only am I fully accepting myself for who I am – the good, the bad, the broken – but also exposing and sharing my story with the world, or at least you guys, the readers. Two things I encourage you to do while reading this, if anything, is to educate yourself and learn from my experiences, but also from the stories of other people in this book.

I am a Muslim, South Asian, East African, 21st-century male, born and raised in Canada, which is quite the diverse background compared to most, I believe. To add to it, I am currently living in Dublin, Ireland, for college for the next five years. I was born with values from all different aspects of my background, some of which include the obvious such as being respectful, honest and ambitious. Some other cultural values I was brought up with were respect your elders, don't let anyone see your emotions, and 'You're a man, you must always be strong'.

Emotionally unstable personality disorder (EUPD), also known as borderline personality disorder (BPD), is a mental illness (while contro-versial) that causes individuals to experience extreme changes in mood that last for several days, affecting your personal relationships. Often, EUPD can be caused by some or all of the following: physical, sexual and emotional abuse, as well as long-term distress as a child. 'Luckily' enough I've experienced all of these, but little did I know I was suffering from EUPD up until a month ago, November 2020. Two months prior, I was being treated for depression and anxiety – both psychologically and pharmacologically. And before that, I had been suffering in silence for as long as I can remember.

I am proud to say that I was brought up in a home that provided me with everything I could ever want and dream of. I have two parents and a brother who love me, even though sometimes it's hard to believe since the idea of love seems so foreign to me. I have a great home and have been provided with opportunities of a lifetime that most wouldn't have, such as travelling and being able to study across the globe. While I am grateful and appreciative of all that my family has given me, unfortunately it wasn't always great. And out of respect for family, I'll choose to keep that between us.

When things started to get really bad, I had just started my second year of college, and amidst a pandemic, to make things worse. I had decided to tell my best friend what was happening, and a question that he asked me stuck in my head, 'When was the last time you felt happy?' And I took a while to answer because I couldn't remember the last time I genuinely felt happy for a long period of time. Sure, I would have moments where I felt great, but those mostly just felt like breaks from the lows. Then, I thought about how I felt during middle school, which brings me to my mental abuse. One thing you should know about me is that I am a very artistic and creative fella, who also enjoys a ton of physical activities, but for some reason my classmates in middle school only focused on the artistic side and labelled me as 'gay'. Now imagine, a little boy whose family is old-fashioned, and who doesn't know the meaning of that word, is told he's gay. Nevertheless, I put on a front, and told myself and everyone around me I wasn't, and it was their choice, and mine, to believe it or not. To say the least, I was confused, and mentally this impacted my life every day.

Little did I know it, Grade 9 was one of the lowest moments of my life. After constantly hearing rumours about my sexuality, I eventually decided to test the theory and meet a random stranger and have sex. I say little did I know it because I did not realise, nor accept that I was raped until a month ago.

Coming to Ireland, I was hoping for a fresh start, and while some did speculate about my sexuality, a whole new problem began – the battle with my mental health. In high school, I was constantly busy and never gave myself much time to breathe, but when I came to university things were different and I had a lot more time to myself and time to overthink. This year was especially bad because of the pandemic, providing me with even more alone time. In September, I began to have suicidal thoughts again, but these were different from the ones I had in high school. As each day passed it got harder to see a future for myself. During the first week of November, I had planned my suicide. I was going to overdose on my anti-depressants; I always told myself if I wanted to kill myself, I'd do it in a way involving the least pain because that's what I am trying to run from. Fortunately, my best friend saved me and took me to the A&E. Two days later I saw Prof. C. and I was diagnosed with EUPD.

Bisexual. Survivor. Anxiety. EUPD.

These are just a few of the words I use to describe my reality. While there is a lot more to my story, what I want to say is this:

Everyone's experience is different and no matter what background/culture you are from mental illness is real and can affect you. And if you are struggling or know someone that is struggling, ask for help! The worst advice and the best advice I can give is have hope; and I use the word worst because I know what it feels like to lose all sense of hope. Create a support system and find the right help that will give you hope, even when you can't find it yourself. If it wasn't for my best friend, I would not be standing here today. And if it wasn't for my diagnosis, I would still be on medications that only worsen my mood and panic attacks. If it wasn't for my support system and my diagnosis, I'd be dead. Having a diagnosis has helped me in many ways, I am now starting to receive the correct help, I am able to see hope for the future, and even though I can't cure this, I can maintain it. I am trying to survive every day, but at least I am trying, and that's what matters the most.

A diagnosis of ADHD in an adult

I was always a boisterous child, one that approached life with energy and enthusiasm. Growing up this was a positive. I found it easy to make friends and had a wide variety of interests.

It was as I got older that it became problematic. As I moved into my later teen years, I was consistently disruptive in school and unreliable when it came to completing assigned tasks in education or part-time jobs. I'll never forget one teacher caveating that our class were occasionally allowed to forget their homework by saying, 'Gareth, this doesn't apply to you, because you never have your homework done'. However, due to a mixture of natural intuition and good fortune I got through my final exams at school. It was when I started at university that things came to a head. My inability to complete assignments and essays would mean that I'd sit end-of-year exams for modules that were nearly mathematically impossible for me to pass. Fail. Fail again. Repeat year.

After several years of this cycle, my mental health had really suffered. I was now 22, my progression in life had ground to a halt and I had lost complete faith in my own abilities.

Thankfully, my family didn't lose faith in me and arranged for me to speak with a psychiatrist. Of course, deep down I knew what the issue was, before it was even suggested. *Had I considered that I might have ADHD?* Of course I had, but I had also allowed myself to believe the nonsense that ADHD wasn't real and was merely an excuse used by people to justify reckless behaviour and poor performance. ADHD, if it was real, was for *other* people. I was an adult at this stage, so surely it would have been detected sooner?

The process for achieving a diagnosis included me undergoing an array of tests. Pinpoint this list of towns on a map. Sure, no problem.

Now do it while this audio beeps in the background. Awful, taunting even. It involved my mother answering a multitude of questions about me growing up. Would Gareth struggle to complete a task if you asked him to? Was his room always messy? Would he lose personal items like wallets and mobile phones? Yes, this was me, all right.

I now had my diagnosis. As part of my treatment plan I was pre-scribed Ritalin. More than the treatment, however, the diagnosis gave me a new-found confidence in myself. It enabled me to accept and explain so many parts of my life that I had previously been unable to. That summer, I arranged to sit the exams for my penultimate year at university. I cannot explain the sensation of actually being able to study after all these years. In some ways I felt cheated that my peers had been able to exist like this for the majority of their lives! I was now able to take notes and complete readings without getting distracted mid-way through and taking an unearned break. I got through the exams and went on to complete my degree.

In the years since then I have relocated to Belgium and work quite a demanding role in the EU institutions. There's no doubt about it though, my ADHD still impacts me, but in both positive and negative ways. My job requires a lot of meeting with people and creativity, as-pects of my character I attribute to my ADHD. It also involves a good degree of organisation, something I continue to struggle with. Overall, it's a condition, like any other, that has to be managed. I decided quite early on that I was going to be very open about my diagnosis and this carried through to the workplace. Of course, disclosure is a very per-sonal choice but I've found that it's good to mention it casually early on so that it doesn't become a bigger issue when I inevitably am unable to manage my tasks properly.

Having spoken with many others with ADHD, I find that the big-gest thing we have in common is our tendency to negatively in-ternalise the ways in which ADHD impacts our lives. We'll spend ages beating ourselves up over not cleaning our apartment or re-neging on that commitment we made to somebody else. I think this is because the ways in which ADHD presents itself can create an impression that somebody is lazy or doesn't care, which gener-ally couldn't be further from the truth. It's difficult to explain why you let somebody down without feeling bad about yourself. But I'm gradually getting better at this.

Receiving my diagnosis, even as an adult, was really a game changer for me. The treatment allowed me to add a degree of structure to my life and get things back on track. On a more personal level, it allowed me to explain behaviours that had previously come across as erratic or unusual.

More than at any other time in human history, our society today requires a high degree of organisation and attention to detail, two things that don't come naturally to people with ADHD. Because of this, my advice to anybody who thinks they might have ADHD is to look into having yourself tested.

11

Disorders Due to Substance Use or Addictive Behaviours

Most people use substances that are not good for their health. Some are legal like alcohol and nicotine, while others are illegal, although there are campaigns to decriminalise or make these legal. The reason they are illegal is because of the damage they do.

Substance abuse and gambling disorder are two common and damaging addictive disorders. The substances that are most commonly abused in Ireland are listed below – alcohol and cannabis are the most commonly abused.

Common substances of abuse

- Alcohol
- Cannabis ('weed', 'hash', 'pot' etc.)
- Hallucinogens, e.g. LSD ('acid'), mescaline, PCP ('angel dust')
- Cocaine ('coke') and crack cocaine
- Amphetamines ('speed'), MDMA ('ecstasy') and ketamine
- Psilocybin ('magic mushrooms')
- Inhalants, e.g. glue
- Opiates, e.g. heroin, methadone
- Benzodiazepines
- Some antidepressants
- Nicotine or tobacco
- Prescription drugs

All of these drugs can cause acute intoxication and can be abused both in the short term or over longer periods. Dependence can follow from repeated use. Once dependence is diagnosed, discontinuing the substance or altering the associated behaviour due to discontinuation symptoms, is very difficult. This process normally requires professional help, community support or, most often, both. In the real world, people frequently abuse multiple drugs simultaneously; for example, someone would combine opiates, hallucinogens and cannabis.

HOW DOES DEPENDENCE MANIFEST?

A behaviour that for many is a harmless indulgence, such as a puff of cannabis or a glass of whiskey, can for some people become habitual, and eventually result in the person finding themselves unable to do without the substance.

The features of substance dependence that you or others will notice are that:

- You have to take the drug in increasing quantities over time to achieve the same effect. So while two glasses of wine would help you to relax initially, one year later four glasses might be required to induce the same state. This is referred to as increasing *tolerance*.

- Despite wanting and trying to cut down, you are unable to, or if you do succeed in cutting down, it is not sustained.

- You devote significant amounts of time trying to procure the drug (particularly when the substance is illegal).

- You spend significant amounts of money buying it (again, especially when the drug is illegal).

- You may have problems with the law. This may be due to debt, or you may be charged with offences such as drink- and drug-driving, theft to finance the habit, or charges of distributing illegal drugs.

- Interpersonal problems with your friends and family may arise, especially if they disapprove of your habit.

- The use of drugs may impact on your ability to hold down employment due to hangovers, tiredness, impaired concentration and focus, and time spent seeking the drugs.

- You will have problems discontinuing the substance, due either to physical withdrawal or to the psychological discomfort that comes with this.
- You may develop psychosis if abusing cannabis, cocaine, amphetamines, LSD or psilocybin.

In the past there was a distinction between psychological and physical dependence. Psychological dependence was believed to be a matter of willpower. There were cravings, to be sure, but it was thought that these could be managed by the person themselves if they were given good support. This was distinguished from those who experienced *physical* symptoms, which were often extremely uncomfortable and even potentially life-threatening during the withdrawal period. Delirium tremens is an example of a physical withdrawal syndrome in those who are alcohol dependent. It causes tremors, high temperature, rapid heart rate, fits, hallucinations that are not frightening but may be amusing, with small images of objects and people (these are known as Lilliputian hallucinations), confusion and, in some, death. It is regarded as a medical emergency and requires inpatient medical treatment.

WHAT CAUSES DEPENDENCE?

The *pharmacological* mechanisms by which these drugs exert their effect on the brain vary with the substance. What they have in common is that the reward system in the brain is triggered by pleasureful activities and this becomes self-reinforcing by means of dopamine. There may be a genetic contribution to this also. This has been demonstrated by studies of twins and also of children adopted because of alcohol problems in their biological families (McGue,1999). The likelihood of alcohol dependence is reduced when one twin has this condition or when adopted children reared by non-alcohol dependent parents are followed up

Dependence does not only have genetic roots, though. Indeed, in many cases, it can originate in childhood trauma, and alcohol and drugs are used to supress painful childhood memories of various types of abuse. A history of sexual, physical or emotional abuse is common in those who abuse substances.

Reward pathway in the brain

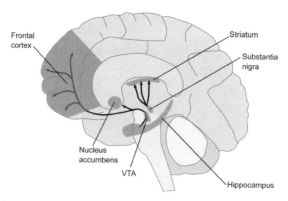

In the brain, dopamine plays an important role in the regulation of reward and movement. As part of the reward pathway, dopamine is manufactured in nerve cell bodies located within the ventral tegmental area (VTA) and is released in the nucleus accumbens and the prefrontal cortex. Its motor functions are linked to a separate pathway, with cell bodies in the substantia nigra that manufacture and release dopamine into the striatum.

A very small portion of substance dependence stems from the manner in which the medical profession has prescribed certain drugs. If a drug is prescribed for prolonged periods or in high doses, there is a chance that the patient will become addicted, even if they have no other risk factors such as a genetic predisposition or a history of abuse. These cases of addiction are not driven primarily by the person's own psychological needs but simply by the physiological effects of substances. This cause of addiction is called *iatrogenic* substance dependence, and it occurs particularly in those prescribed opiates or benzodiazepines for physical reasons, e.g. chronic pain.

PSYCHIATRIC COMPLICATIONS OF SUBSTANCE MISUSE

The range of psychiatric complications varies from drug to drug:

Mood changes

Serious fluctuations in mood can occur in those taking cocaine, amphetamines, MDMA, benzodiazepines, LSD and alcohol. In some, particularly in relation to withdrawal from cocaine, a period in hospital may even be required for reasons of safety, since suicidal ideation and profound depression can accompany discontinuation of these drugs or their abuse. Antidepressants are not required unless the symptoms persist after the drugs have been excreted by the body a few days later.

Induced psychosis

Drug-induced psychoses are a group of conditions caused by some drugs. They usually begin quickly and subside after the drug has been excreted from the body. These episodes last a few hours to a few days. The drugs mainly causing this are illegal ones, and cannabis, amphetamines and LSD are particularly problematic.

The symptoms of drug-induced psychosis often consist of delusions, often of a paranoid nature, believing that others are wanting to harm them, and/or hallucinations. Auditory hallucinations – hearing voices when there is nobody about and nothing to explain them – are the most common symptom. Tactile hallucinations – unexplained sensations under the skin – are common with cocaine in particular, and so this symptom has come to be called the 'cocaine bug'. All these are very frightening experiences for the person and for those close to them. The paranoid delusions may be particularly intense and can result in violent behaviour.

Sometimes these symptoms do not resolve even when the drug is no longer in the body, and psychiatric consultation or hospital admission may be required along with medication to alleviate the symptoms. If the symptoms continue despite this, the diagnosis will change from drug-induced psychosis to a longer-term condition such as schizophrenia or delusional disorder (for these conditions, see Chapter 8).

In addition to causing psychotic episodes, illicit drugs often destabilise and trigger psychiatric *relapses* in those with pre-existing illnesses such as bipolar disorder or schizophrenia. It is thus of paramount importance that if you are diagnosed with any prior psychotic illness you steer well clear of these drugs, even in small quantities.

A different kind of psychosis is diagnosed when there is an underlying physical illness causing the symptoms. This may be pneumonia, brain injury or a host of other physical conditions. The symptoms are due to a reduction in the supply of oxygen to the brain.

Another pattern of psychotic symptoms occurs when there are specifically focused psychotic symptoms as a consequence of long-standing substance abuse, such as paranoia or pathological jealousy, also called *Othello syndrome,* derived from Othello's murderous jealousy of his wife in the eponymous Shakespearean tragedy.

Alcoholic hallucinosis is another recognised condition, in which only a voice or voices are heard and nothing else explains them. This occurs during or after a period of heavy alcohol consumption. The symptom may improve over time with treatment, but this does not always happen and sometimes the hallucinosis persists.

Cognitive impairment

Cognitive impairment, a term for impairment in memory and other brain functions, may be due to alcohol-related brain disease. Sometimes the person may fill in gaps in their memory with stories that are manifestly false. This is called 'confabulation' and has also been termed 'Korsakoff's psychosis', after the man who originally named it. So the person might convincingly tell you that they were in Dublin shopping with a cousin last week and that they bought a new coat and shoes, when in fact they were at home with their husband in County Cork where they live and had not been shopping anywhere. The stories may sometimes be more elaborate, such as going to the President's house with a group of visitors last year and having lunch with him!

Harm during pregnancy

The unborn child may be affected if the mother abuses alcohol during pregnancy, particularly in the first three months. Foetal alcohol syndrome, as this is called, is a condition in the baby that causes brain damage, deformities of the joints and slow physical growth. There may be facial abnormalities, heart defects and visual or hearing problems. These are not reversible, so it is imperative that pregnant women do not drink. The use of illicit drugs may have broadly similar effects, although the research is less conclusive. It is strongly advised that pregnant women err on the side of caution and refrain from all substances during pregnancy. Even aside from this syndrome, all illegal drugs increase the risk of stillbirth, and newborn infants may experience *infant withdrawal symptoms* from substances. Again it is important to refrain from non-prescribed drugs during pregnancy. Shamefully, Ireland has the third highest rate of foetal alcohol syndrome in the world, after South Africa and Croatia ((Lange et al., 2017), pointing to the necessity for action on this.

PSYCHOSOCIAL AND RELATIONSHIP IMPACT OF SUBSTANCE MISUSE

The effects of substance misuse on a person's children are significant (Velleman et al., 2016) and can lead to serious problems for them in later life. The most obvious effect is the emotional deprivation from a parent who was effectively absent, and physical and sexual abuse are also ever-present risks. Other problems will arise indirectly from poverty,and unemployment, and witnessing violence between parents. Legal problems stemming from violence and drink-driving are common in both adult and child victims of substance misuse. Many of those who abuse substances lack insight, and either wilfully or unknowingly convince themselves that these are harmless.

TREATMENT

Detoxification and aftercare

During withdrawal from drugs many will experience cravings. These cravings are not in themselves dangerous, but they are very uncomfortable and may hinder the withdrawal process, possibly resulting in relapse. There is no simple answer to craving during withdrawal apart from support from others. It is the physical symptoms that can be most dangerous (Fearon et al., 2017).

* **Alcohol dependence**

In respect of alcohol the withdrawal symptoms consist of tremors, sweating, feeling anxious, nausea, vomiting, high temperature and sweating. Fits, racing heart, confusion and visual hallucinations (with the objects frequently being small in size or funny) are serious and require urgent medical attention. This is known as the 'DTs', or delirium tremens (see p.197). By taking benzodiazepines (e.g. chlordiazepoxide, marketed as Librium) in high enough doses during the withdrawal period, along with multivitamins, alcohol withdrawal symptoms can be reduced. If multivitamins are not prescribed, neurological problems involving the eyes, along with poor memory and efforts to fill in memory gaps with false stories due to brain damage, may follow. Symptoms like persistent hallucinations or paranoia may persist after withdrawal.

For alcohol dependence, treatment lies mainly with primary care (GPs) and continuing community care through the HSE drugs and alcohol service. The withdrawal during the initial phase lasts about two weeks and the cravings are intense, but there is no treatment for this. Some may require inpatient treatment for detoxification, particularly as doing so at home, even with psychological help, has been unsuccessful in the past.

There are different practices around the country among psychiatrists regarding detoxification. Some will not admit a person who needs detoxification to a psychiatric unit because of fear that delirium tremens may occur and a belief that outpatient approaches are best. Others will admit the person and commence the detoxification process, and if the DTs develop the person will then be transferred to the medical team. This is a serious condition with a mortality of about 15%.

Following detoxification, the person should then obtain support in the community. This includes attending self-help groups such as Alcoholics Anonymous or alcohol treatment programmes run by the HSE to assist people in remaining abstinent. Psychological counselling is the mainstay of treatment after the withdrawal phase. Others attend rehab residential programmes to assist.

Sometimes medication such as disulfiram (Antabuse) deters people from drinking by inducing nausea when the tablets are taken with alcohol.

Those who say they are depressed after a period of detoxification should have a period of watchful waiting before consideration is given to antidepressants. Some experience low mood secondary to the impact of alcohol on the brain or as a result of psychosocial problems associated with alcohol. Once alcohol is discontinued the improvement in mood occurs in a few weeks without antidepressants.

• **Benzodiazepines**
Those taking benzodiazepines for more than about six weeks may experience physical symptoms of anxiety as well as epileptic fits if they discontinue the medications suddenly. By using these medications in the

lowest dose to achieve symptom relief, and only as needed rather than regularly, this can be avoided. If you have a benzodiazepine problem your GP should prescribe a long-acting preparation and then taper the dose at a speed that is comfortable for you. This may happen over a period of weeks and inpatient detoxification is seldom required.

- **Opiates**

Opiates such as heroin or morphine require slow tapering also. Many opiate abusers are changed from their primary addictive drug to methadone and the dose of this is reduced gradually. The discontinuation symptoms are collectively referred to as 'cold turkey' because the person feels cold, with goose bumps, is nauseated, has shivers and a runny nose, experiences joint pains and vomits. This is not fatal (although the person may often feel as if they're about to die), but if the person resumes the opiate after a period of abstinence their tolerance for the drug will have dropped. They might not realise that their tolerance has lowered, though, and a tragically common story in Ireland is of a person returning straight to their old dosage level after a period off the sauce and accidentally killing themselves by overdosing.

- **Other drugs**

Most other drugs of abuse do not require any specific intervention for withdrawal since the symptoms are mainly concerned with craving and low mood. For these, supportive measures and psychological interventions, including motivational interviewing, are the most commonly used. Cocaine, in particular, is associated with a severe drop in mood after it has been stopped. Concentration and fatigue are common, as are increased appetite, nightmares, exhaustion and suicidal thoughts (there is a real danger that these thoughts will be carried out).

Nicotine withdrawal is managed by GPs and is rarely dealt with by psychiatrists. If you have tried to stop smoking on your own without success, you should consult your GP. People also find support groups helpful in maintaining their resolve.

PRACTICAL CONSIDERATIONS

On the ground, the provision of treatment for those with substance use disorders varies enormously. The HSE has a dedicated group of services and therapists. Inpatient treatment may be required for alcohol and opiate detoxification, but for the most part treatment is offered in the community. This may be done by psychiatrists, but in the case of opiates, such as heroin, it is done by GPs and addiction specialists.

Residential care is an option post-detoxification for those who previously abused alcohol or opiates. There is a number of such units in Ireland, which can be accessed through the HSE or through charities. Continuing therapy lasts for several months and is psychologically based. For many recovering addicts religious faith is important and one centre in Ireland (Tiglin) offers a spiritual/religious approach combined with the standard psychological techniques.

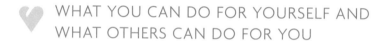

WHAT YOU CAN DO FOR YOURSELF AND WHAT OTHERS CAN DO FOR YOU

- Remaining abstinent from alcohol or drugs cannot be done alone. Ask family/friends for help and join a support group.
- If your loved one is abusing alcohol, Al-Anon will help you to deal with this.
- Do not believe those who tell you cannabis is harmless.
- Do not tell yourself that a line of cocaine is OK after dinner with friends.
- Do not think you will be OK taking illegal drugs from time to time.
- Sometimes benzodiazepines are necessary in the short term, but take them with caution.
- Illicit drug-taking will only be fun for a while.
- Do not try to persuade a person who has become psychotic due to drugs that their experience of voices or of delusions is their imagination.

BIBLIOGRAPHY

Farren, Conor. *Overcoming Alcohol Misuse: A 28-Day Guide.* Dublin: Kite Books. 2011.

Lange, S., Probst, C., Gmel, G. et al. 'Global Prevalence of fetal alcohol spectrum among children and youth. A systematic review and meta-analysis'. *JAMA Pediatrics.* Doi:10.1001/jamapediatrics2017.1919. 2017.

McGue, M. 'The behavioral genetics of alcoholism'. *Current Directions in Psychological Science* 8:109–15. 1999.

Velleman, Richard and Templeton, Lorna J. 'Impact of parents' substance misuse on children: an update'. *BJPsych Advances*, vol. 22, 108–11. 2016.

USEFUL RESOURCES

Anderson, Rolande. *Living with a Problem Drinker. Your Survival Guide.* Boston, MA: Sheldon Press. 2010.

Brand, Russell. *Recovery, Freedom from our Addictions.* London: Picador. 2018.

www.problemgambling.ie

Mayo Clinic. Compulsive Gambling – Mayo Clinic. Mayoclinic.org. N.p. 2016 web

Rutland Centre for Gambling Rehabilitation. 01-4946358; or info@rutlandcentre.ie

HSE Drugs and Alcohol helpline: helpline@hse.ie

Al Anon Information Services, 5 Capel Street, Dublin DO1TH76.

Narcotics Anonymous Ireland, 14 Kevin Street Upper, Portobello, Dublin. 01-6728000.

Addiction – listening and opening up

This is my story of how my mental health was affected and led to addiction and suicide attempts.

My earliest memory of a change in my life was when I suddenly found myself coming from a broken home; father was an alcoholic and spent most of his days in the pub – he would come home with no money and fight with my mother. This is where my story began.

After all the abuse my mother took off him, she eventually threw him out and left herself with two young kids. Back in them days women not standing by their men was not to be seen. My mother could not take it any more. This meant I had to go to school at a very young age and lie about having a dad at home. Because of this I quickly learned how to lie and not feel that I was doing anything wrong because lying was my defence mode to keep myself safe. I carried this with me all the way to my adult years. Little did I know at the time my mental health was impacted by the hurt and sadness.

As I grew up as a teenager, I was mad into sports (football) so this kept me away from trouble, but I always had this thing inside me where I did not care any more, why would I, I fought my way through life on my own. It was when I was 18–21 I started to drink with friends, I always wanted to be the person that got drunk the most and had to be carried home, this was a false persona of the person I really was. I thought this new me would make my life better. I also had a thing in my mind I was on my own in life so nobody told me what to do or how much I could drink. Then came drugs and gambling, where I was also dabbling in class A and spending money I did not have in the bookies.

This became my life. I thought this is the way a young man should live his life. I lived this unhappy life right through my 20s, destroying my mental health with depression and multiple suicide thoughts. It was when I had my children it gave me a glimpse of what life should be about and where I wanted to be in life, but as addiction and mental health go very well together it was tough to break the cycle.

Then came one day when the build-up of years of depression finally got the better of me. I told my partner to bring the kids down to the supermarket. I was planning to take my life. I sat there and cried like a baby, fighting with myself whether to take my life or not. I just wanted the pain to stop. When I was about to do the unthinkable, I received a WhatsApp message from my mother with just 'love you' written in the comments. This message was enough to knock me off track. As I sat there crying, my partner walked back into the house with my children and they both ran to me and gave me a big hug. Everything was out in the open and I felt a big weight come off my shoulders. I spoke to a friend and he recommended a rehabilitation centre. I knew if I tried to get help through the community, I would end up back where I started. So I entered a rehab centre at 38 years old.

I really wanted to change my life this time and I was really focused. After all, I did leave my family behind, which was the hardest decision I ever had to make. I taught myself some skills that would change my life for ever. For a person that never listened to anybody I started to listen. I opened my heart up to faith, something that I never done before. I heard somebody saying one day there are things in life you should always have – RESPECT and HONESTY. If you can't respect yourself you can't respect others, and if you can't be honest with yourself you can't be honest with others.

Today I am a happy man, loving life with my partner and children. I am currently learning a new language, studying IT and volunteering to help people in my situation. it's been nearly two years since I had a drink, took drugs or gambled, and my mental health is stable. This was all done without any medication, some hard work, faith and allowing myself to be the person I always wanted to be – kind, fun-loving and caring. That in itself is freedom

When I look back now and think of the timing of that message there must be a God, because if that message was sent a few seconds later I might not be here to tell this story.

12

Eating Disorders, Dementia and Psychosexual Disorders

This chapter deals with three groups of disorders, all important but not long enough in themselves to warrant a full chapter each.

EATING DISORDERS

We think of eating disorders as related to lifestyle and the modern world. But even in the 12th century there were records of women fasting to overcome their gluttony. Anorexia mirabilis (miraculous lack of appetite) was the name given to this phenomenon. The women who practised it were thought to be possessed of supernatural holiness and some were regarded as saints. So when Dr Richard Morton, an English physician, first described a wasting condition in 1689, it was nothing new. There was no further documentation of cases until some 200 years later, in 1873, when another English physician, Sir William Gull, coined the term 'anorexia nervosa'. He described a series of cases around the same time that a French physician, Ernest Charles Lessing, also identified a similar pattern in some of his patients. Anorexia nervosa is the least common eating disorder, but it is the one with which the public is most familiar. It is overwhelmingly more common in females than males by a ratio of 5 or even 10 to 1, but it affects fewer than 1% of females.

More recently, in 1979, *bulimia nervosa* was described by another British doctor, the late Professor Gerald Russell (Russell, 1979), who was known to many of us in the psychiatric profession and was viewed with great affection. He described the condition as an irresistible urge to over-eat followed by self-induced vomiting or purging to compensate for this. There may also be excessive exercise. There is preoccupation with weight and shape as in anorexia nervosa. The person may have food fads and an extreme dietary regime. So, there are behaviours that are found in anorexia nervosa interspersed with bingeing and compensatory activities. Russell that believed bulimia nervosa was a variant of anorexia nervosa and that it was a culture-bound condition linked to modern life. Unlike those with anorexia nervosa, those with bulimia nervosa tended to be heavier and many continued to menstruate. They often suffered severe depressive symptoms. This is the second most common eating disorder, present in 2–3% of the population.

Binge eating disorder is another recognised eating disorder. It was first described in 1959 by American psychiatrist Albert Stunkard, but it was not accepted as a psychiatric disorder until 2013. Binge eating disorder is characterised by regularly eating to excess even when not hungry, feeling disgusted with oneself for this and eating alone because of embarrassment at being seen to consume so much. The person feels a lack of control of these episodes. Unlike bulimia nervosa the binges are not usually followed by attempts to compensate for the over-eating by purging. While it has only recently come to psychiatric attention, binge eating disorder is calculated as affecting 3–4% of the population. It goes without saying that those who occasionally binge do not have the disorder.

The causes of eating disorders are not fully understood. Some of those affected have a history of childhood sexual abuse, or of obesity in childhood, for which they were bullied. The perfectionism and drive found in many of those with these disorders have also been considered, as has the cultural ideal, in many countries, of women as slim. Indeed, one of the explanations for the very low rate of eating disorders in the Arab world, especially anorexia nervosa, is that Arab cultures do not have the same ideal of women as thin. However, the rate of the disorder is rising in many of these countries, though this may be attributable to changing socio-cultural attitudes to body size and shape.

HOW DO THOSE WITH EATING DISORDERS PRESENT TO THE DOCTOR?

Concerns about dieting and anorexia nervosa are not usually raised by those affected because they do not accept that their eating habits or weight changes are a problem. Yet, family, friends or teachers will often be aware of unhealthy dietary habits, particularly dietary restriction. Anorexia nervosa usually begins in adolescence or early adulthood, and it can extend well into the adult years.

The body mass index (BMI) is a measure of the appropriateness of a person's weight. It can easily be calculated by dividing the person's weight (in kilograms) by their height (in metres squared). This is only an estimate, though, and some people, especially if they have a high muscle mass, can seem to be overweight when in fact they are perfectly healthy. It would be worth discussing your weight with your doctor or with a dietetics expert if you have concerns about it. Further details about BMI measurements are shown below.

Body Mass Index (BMI)

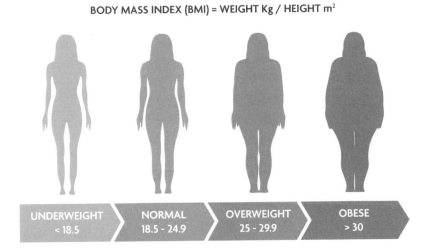

BODY MASS INDEX (BMI) = WEIGHT Kg / HEIGHT m²

UNDERWEIGHT	NORMAL	OVERWEIGHT	OBESE
< 18.5	18.5 - 24.9	25 - 29.9	> 30

Among those with anorexia nervosa the weight loss is self-induced, usually by avoiding foods that the person deems to be fattening, or by self-inducing vomiting, or by purging using laxatives. These two methods are known as *restricting* and *purging* respectively. Vigorous exercise and sometimes even diuretic medication (to reduce the fluid in tissue cells) may also be used. There is distortion of the body image so that the person sees themselves as fat rather than a normal weight or even underweight. This false self-perception increases as thinness increases, and for this reason as weight decreases dieting will increase in tandem.

The obvious symptoms are food restriction either in quantity or in the type of food eaten, amenorrhoea (loss of menstruation), cold hands and feet, dry skin, hair loss, the presence of fine downy hair on the body (called lanugo). Loss of fat is obvious to others. There are physiological signs too, such as low blood pressure, slowing of the heart rate, anaemia, a reduction in white cells, low blood sugar, low potassium and low chloride. Some of these, such as low potassium, are life threatening. Increased levels of growth hormone and of cortisol are also found, and there may be visible tooth decay due to the physical effects of vomiting on teeth. Among men, instead of amenorrhoea, anorexia nervosa may lead to loss of sexual interest (loss of libido) or impotence (difficulty achieving and maintaining an erection).

Many of those with anorexia nervosa are sent initially to an endocrine disorder specialist since their symptoms are also found in those with certain gland problems. In anorexia nervosa they will rectify if food intake improves. There are two types of anorexia nervosa: the restricting type and the purging type, although both can occur together. The weight loss is noticeable and the person may even look emaciated. In this it differs from the weight loss that accompanies other psychiatric conditions, such as depression or anxiety. It is very common for those who suffer with anorexia nervosa to deny that they have it; this can, of course, delay treatment, with serious consequences. Bulimia nervosa and binge eating disorder are more likely to be diagnosed early in the course of the condition, since the person usually presents with weight gain.

Eating disorders are best treated with psychological interventions. There is some evidence that bulimia nervosa responds to high-dose SSRI antidepressants. However, these should not be used on their own: they normally only work in combination with psychological treatment. Family therapy may also be necessary for those with anorexia nervosa as they often exhibit strained family relationships. Sometimes it may be necessary for the doctor to obtain a court order to feed a young person who is dying of starvation due to anorexia nervosa. For the person and their family this can be extremely distressing. In some instances the courts have supported forced feeding.

DEMENTIA AND OTHER ORGANIC BRAIN CONDITIONS

Dementia is a term used to describe a general loss of memory, language and other cognitive abilities. These are severe enough to interfere with daily living. Dementia is not just the result of normal ageing. Some amount of forgetfulness is normal as we age: we may find it difficult to remember simple things, such as what we need to get out of the cupboard, or where we have put our keys. This is distinct from dementia, though: those with dementia suffer disturbance of many brain functions, not just memory (although memory is often the most prominent loss in the early stages). Those with dementia may lose orientation in relation to where they are, or what year or time of day it is. Comprehension of language, decisions involving judgement, and personality features can all also be compromised. This is because there is widespread damage to areas in the brain that are crucial to day-to-day functioning. As such, in addition to memory impairment, those with dementia will have difficulties in managing their day-to-day lives. Ovens may be left on, saucepans may be left to burn, and the person may forget to eat. They are prone to falls and they may wander from home and get lost. They may also be prone to financial exploitation by predators, and may be victims of 'elder abuse', including assault. Sometimes the onset of early dementia may be indicated by a presentation with depression, anxiety or psychosis for the first time in later adulthood.

About one in 20 people over the age of 75 will have dementia, and this increases to one in five among those over the age of 80. Dementia can also occur in those under the age of 65 (this is known as early-onset dementia), but this is much less common. It has been found in certain sportsmen, particularly rugby players and boxers, possibly as a result of head injuries.

TYPES OF DEMENTIA

There are several kinds of dementia:

- *Alzheimer's disease* is the most common. There is the gradual onset of memory impairment and decline in other functions mentioned already. When it occurs in those under 65 it is called presenile dementia. The causes of dementia are multifaceted and it is believed that genes contribute in part to the onset of dementia. Environmental factors such as high blood pressure and obesity have also been identified. In some cases, there is no reason that we can discern. Post-mortem studies have shown particular abnormalities in brain tissue, though, and these are called neurofibrillary tangles.

- The second type of dementia is *vascular dementia*, and this affects approximately 30% of people with a dementing condition. This sometimes has an abrupt onset, followed by a levelling-off of the symptoms, followed in turn by a further deterioration – as though it were happening in a stepwise pattern.

- *Lewy body dementia* is a condition that affects about 10% of those with dementia and it is associated with Parkinson's disease–type symptoms. The person may experience slowness in walking, tremors and visual hallucinations (i.e. seeing people and objects that are actually not present). Memory may fluctuate considerably and can do so very rapidly – in the course of a few hours. It can be interspersed with periods of well-being and alertness.

- Finally, there is have *frontotemporal dementia*. This disorder is unusual in its presentation and it can sometimes affect those under the age of 60. In this group, personality change, difficulty speaking, impaired concentration and developing rituals that resemble OCD (see Chapter 6) are the most significant initial complaints. Memory loss occurs, but it is not an early symptom and instead occurs late in the condition.

Dementia is diagnosed by taking a history from the person and their relative. A clinical psychologist can carry out tests of memory to establish the diagnosis and a brain scan can also assist. However, there may be evidence of dementia clinically and on psychological testing before it is visible in a brain scan.

TREATING DEMENTIA

Unfortunately, there is no cure for dementia. Basic management of those with dementia involves making sure the person avoids daytime napping. They should be given social simulation by meeting with other people. This also means that they should not be sitting in front of a TV for long periods. Exercise should also be encouraged. Their carers should take responsibility for any treatments they receive, and they should be advised that it is best to begin drug treatments for memory early in the illness. Practical help needs to be provided for the family, such as a home help, respite for holidays and, ultimately, nursing home care.

The use of antipsychotics to relieve agitation or hallucinations should be avoided. Those with dementia have an increased sensitivity to these medications so they may have side effects, such as drowsiness, at lower doses than usual.

Treatment is with medications that will increase the availability of certain neurochemicals that are lost due to the dementing process. These medications are mainly used for Alzheimer's disease, but may be effective in other types of dementia also. They can improve memory but they will not alter the course of the disease, which is progressive.

If the person is being treated by a specialist, the treatment they receive here should be linked to the person's GP. The person will probably wish to know their diagnosis and, if so, this should be done in conjunction with the person's GP and family. The information should be given in a sensitive manner. Possible issues to be discussed are listed on p.216. This should happen in the early stages of the illness while the person has the ability to understand their relevance.

> ### Discussion topics in early dementia
>
> - The diagnosis and likely course
>
> - The person's ability to drive
>
> - Enduring power of attorney – this would nominate a person to take care of their financial affairs should they no longer be able to do so.
>
> - Advance directive – decisions regarding treatment at a later stage in the disease, e.g. antibiotics for infection, resuscitation, treatment for new physical conditions. Should be retested regularly.
>
> - Making a will.

Those who suffer severe depressive illness (see Chapter 7) can appear to have dementia. This is due to the poor concentration and apathy that accompany depressive illness. This is called *depressive pseudodementia* and it clears up with treatment of the depression.

DELIRIUM

Delirium, also called an *acute confusional state,* occurs suddenly, lasting a period of a few hours or at most a few days. It presents with changes in consciousness leading to drowsiness or agitation, combined with restlessness. The person will be disorientated, unable to tell the time, where they are, or who you or others well known to them are. There may also be changes in perception such that the person may believe that they see an object or a person when there is nobody present or nothing to explain it. These are called visual hallucinations. Sometimes the person may also have paranoid delusions. Anxiety, fear and aggression may accompany the delirium. Common causes include infections, and brain trauma due to injury or a stroke. Delirium may occur shortly after surgery or after an epileptic seizure. More common-or-garden causes are pain, constipation and dehydration. Any medical condition can cause delirium, though it is most common in the conditions mentioned. It can occur in any age group but older people are more susceptible, particularly if there is an underlying dementia or if they have visual or hearing impairment. The important thing is that delirium is short-lived and a full recovery is usual.

If you are caring for somebody at home who is experiencing delirium, it is important to encourage them to eat and take fluids. Somebody should stay with them to keep them safe because there is a danger of wandering in this confused state. Make sure that you talk to them and repeat things. At night, keep a lamp alight beside the bed so that they can see what they are doing. This will reduce the risk of misinterpreting shadows as people coming into the room. This condition can be managed at home provided the cause is known (e.g. if it is simply a symptom of a chest infection). If not, then a period in hospital for investigation of the cause will be needed. You can be of great assistance to the treating doctor since they will need to know what the person's baseline was – this will help them in determining whether this is worsening dementia or is really delirium

Treatment of delirium rests with treating the underlying cause. So, for instance, antibiotics will be needed when the delirium is due to an infection. If hallucinations, paranoid delusions or marked agitation are present, then antipsychotic medication may be necessary until the condition settles. Some people with underlying dementia may be excessively sensitive to these, and benzodiazepines such as Valium may be more appropriate replacements. The exception to this is *delirium tremens*, which often happens after surgery due to the sudden cessation of alcohol. For this sort of delirium, the treatment is specific to that condition; benzodiazepines and multivitamins are the standard treatment (Schuckit, 2014) (see Chapter 11). Physicians in this instance are likely to involve psychiatrists because of the treatment required following discharge. For all other sorts of delirium, though, psychiatrists are seldom called, since geriatricians and other medics are familiar with managing this condition. For those being treated at home, the family doctor will be involved. Most people make a complete recovery from delirium.

CONDITIONS RELATED TO SEXUAL HEALTH

A number of sexual disorders are recognised in psychiatry. Most people with these conditions tend to be referred by their GPs to sexual health clinics rather than to psychiatrists. Nonetheless, they may occur secondary to some psychiatric disorders or as a result of medication, and in that context people are seen by psychiatrists. Some may also be referred for investigation of sexual behaviours when a crime is alleged to have been committed and a psychiatric cause has to be ruled out.

Sexual disorders are grouped into three main categories (Reed et al., 2020).

1. Sexual dysfunctions

The first, referred to as *sexual dysfunctions*, includes five broad diagnoses.

Sexual dysfunction disorders

- Sexual desire and arousal dysfunctions
- Orgasmic dysfunctions
- Ejaculatory dysfunctions
- Other unspecified conditions
- Sexual pain-penetration disorder

These conditions may be present as part of a psychiatric condition. For instance, loss of libido, in both men and women, occurs in depressive illness. Hypersexuality may occur at the manic pole of bipolar disorder. Alcohol or other substance dependence and antidepressants may cause erectile dysfunction. These are helped by treating the underlying condition in the usual way. However, those with erectile dysfunction can also be speedily helped by taking sildenafil (also called Viagra) or tadalafil (also called Cialis). Sexual pain disorder was previously called vaginismus, and this requires a specialist psychosexual therapist. The prognosis is good. It may sometimes occur in the context of having experienced sexual abuse.

2. Gender identity

The second is the group related to gender identity. The psychiatric condition relating to a feeling that one's gender is not the gender one is 'given' or that one was 'assigned at birth' has two names: gender incongruence (ICD-11) and gender dysphoria (DSM-5). This is the condition that transgender ('trans') people have. Many think that it is inappropriate for gender incongruence to be a medical condition, and it is likely that it will be removed entirely from the psychiatric classifications in due course, just as homosexuality was in 1974. According to Reed (2020), though, gender incongruence is retained so that transgender people can access mental health services that otherwise might not be available to them if the condition were removed, so there are at least practical reasons for retaining it for the moment. Gender incongruence, particularly in children and adolescents, has become controversial in recent years, due in part to the massive surge in numbers coming forward, particularly young women, many of whom are on the autistic spectrum and have other significant co-occurring conditions such as depressive illness and anxiety disorder. The controversy is fuelled by the use of puberty-blocking drugs and cross-sex hormonal treatment. A recent High Court decision in England questioned the practice of using these drugs on children and adolescents under the age of 16, due to issues relating to the capacity of minors to consent to treatment. For those between 16 and 18 the judgement suggested that a court order may be necessary to allow such interventions to proceed. Those who request gender reassignment surgery, whether they are children, adolescents or adults, are seen by psychiatrists as part of this process, but until the surge in recent years among children and adolescents, such evaluations were rare. Some children here are treated in Ireland, but many are referred to the services in England. Adults in Ireland receive hormonal treatments but travel abroad for gender reassignment. The prevalence of adult gender incongruence in Europe is one per 30,000 adult natal males and one per 100,000 natal females (Memom and Xiong, 2019)

The term *transvestism*, dressing in the clothes of the opposite gender so as to experience sexual arousal or the enjoy the experience of simulating the opposite sex without any wish for a permanent sex change, has been recommended for deletion from the ICD–11. According to Reed et al. (2020), this behaviour will no longer be regarded as a psychiatric disorder since it is private in nature and is thought to have no public health relevance.

3. Disorders of sexual preference

The third group relates to disorders of *sexual preference*, known as *paraphilic disorders* (listed below). These conditions involve:

a) a sustained, focused and intense pattern of sexual arousal – as manifested by persistent sexual thoughts, fantasies, urges or behaviours

b) others whose age or status renders them unwilling or unable to consent (e.g. prepubescent children, an unsuspecting individual being viewed through a window, an animal);

c) that the individual, having acted on these thoughts, fantasies or urges, or is markedly distressed by them (Reed et al., 2020).

People with this group of conditions are seen by psychiatrists most often in the context of legal proceedings. A person engaging in such behaviour for the first time will often be referred to a psychiatrist to establish whether the behaviour is driven by a mental illness or by a physical change to the brain, such as dementia.

Paraphilic disorders

- **Exhibitionistic disorder** – exposing genitalia to strangers for shock or sexual pleasure without inviting closer contact

- **Voyeuristic disorder** – watching others engaging in sexual activity or other intimacies such as undressing, using the bathroom

- **Paedophilic disorder** – a sexual preference for children or adolescents

- **Coercive sexual sadism disorder** – a preference for engaging in sexual behaviour involving pain and/or humiliation, such as bondage

- **Frotteuristic disorder** – rubbing against people for sexual stimulation in crowded places, reportedly the most common paraphilia; reported in 7–10% of the population

- **Others** – necrophilia (sexual attraction to corpses), fetishism (sexual attraction to non-living objects)

Paedophilia is the most frequently discussed paraphilic condition. The prevalence is unknown but most sexual offenders against children are men, with females accounting for between 0.4–4% of convicted sexual offenders.

It is defined in psychiatry as a primary or exclusive sexual attraction to pre-pubescent children (i.e. children under the age of 13). It is diagnosed only when the person is over the age of 16, and five or more years older than the child who is the target. The attraction to children emerges during the teenage years. The term ephebophilia was originally used in the late 19th century to describe attraction to those in the adolescent age group, but this is not a psychiatrically accepted concept. It is unclear what term best de-scribes sexual attraction to this age group ('pederasty' is another possibility with some currency). The term paedophilia is used more loosely in day-to-day language to describe somebody who engages in a sexual act with those below the age of 16 or 18, or for whom the attraction may not be a primary one (i.e. for those who are also or even mostly attracted to adults).

Some paedophiles are only attracted to children, while others are at-tracted to both adults and children. It is more common among men than women by a ratio of 4:1. Usually the paedophile is known to the child – a step-parent, a grandparent, or a person in authority such as a teacher, clergyman or sports coach.

The causes are not clear, and although some studies have identified brain abnormalities, these are far from definitive. Others point to the con-tribution of factors impacting on the child *in utero*. It is also the case that many were themselves abused as children, although this is now disputed.

The relationship between viewing child pornography and molesting children is unclear. Some studies show a clear link, with one leading to the other (Sher and Carey, 2007), while others disagree (Endrass and Urbaniok, 2009).

Treatment for paedophilia is with psychotherapy, and in some coun-tries, drugs that reduce libido or that replace testosterone with a drug simi-lar to oestrogens can be prescribed. Paedophilia cannot be cured, but some paedophiles can be assisted in managing their urges, and this is more likely to occur if the person seeks treatment rather than having it imposed by legal fiat. These interventions should be combined with strictly limited ac-cess to children, and close supervision should be ensured. If convicted, the person's name will be on the sexual offences register.

WHAT YOU CAN DO FOR YOURSELF AND WHAT OTHERS CAN DO FOR YOU

Eating disorders
- If you're concerned about your weight, discuss it with your doctor.
- If a family member has an eating disorder, do not get into arguments with them about food.

Dementia and delirium
- If you have a family member with dementia ensure you have time for yourself: apply for a carer or home help to assist.
- Ensure that the person continues to read and listen to the radio and gets mental stimulation.
- Ensure that the person gets exercise.

Conditions related to sexual health
- Difficulties related to sexual function do not disappear – help is needed for these. However, help is also available, and medical professionals will listen to you non-judgementally.
- If somebody has uncertainty about their sexuality, this should be discussed with a professional.
- If you suspect or are aware of a sexual crime against a child you *must* report this to the Gardaí or to Child and Family Services (Tusla).

BIBLIOGRAPHY

Endrass, J. and Urbaniok, F. 'The consumption of Internet child pornography and violent and sex offending'. *BMC Psychiatry*. 9 (43): 43. 2009. doi:10.1186/1471–244X–9–43. PMC 2716325. PMID 19602221.

Memom, M. A. and Xiong, G. L. 'Gender Dysphoria: Practice Essentials'. emedicine.medscape.com. 2019

Reed, D. M., Drescher, J., Krueger, R. et al. 'Disorders related to sexuality and gender identity in the ICD-11: revising the ICD-10 classification based on current scientific evidence, best clinical practices, and human rights considerations'. *World Psychiatry*. 15, 205–21. 2016.

Russell, G. F. M. 'Bulimia nervosa: an ominous variant of anorexia nervosa'. *Psychological Medicine*. 9. 429–48. 1979.

Schuckit, M. A. S. 'Recognition and Management of Withdrawal Delirium Tremens (Delirium Tremens)', *New England Journal of Medicine*. 317: 2109–113. 2014.

Sher, J. and Carey, B. 'Debate on Child Pornography's Link To Molesting'. *New York Times*. 19 July 2007.

USEFUL RESOURCES

Eating Disorders

Bodywhys support service 01-2107906

Lois Bridges Eating Disorders Treatment Centre. 01-8396147 for information (this is for information and not an endorsement).

Brown, Harriet. *Brave Girl Eating: A Family's Struggle with Anorexia*. New York, NY: William Morrow Paperbacks. 2011.

Dementia and delirium

https://www.alzheimers.org.uk/get-support/publications-factsheets/caring-person-dementia-practical-guide: 18

Robins, Peter V. *Is it Alzheimers? Answers to your most pressing questions about memory loss*. Baltimore, MD: Johns Hopkins uUiversity Press. 2020.

Psychosexual Health

A Help Guide for Sexual Problems – causes, signs, treatment options and sources of support. https://www.harleytherapy.co.uk/sexual-problems-help-guide.htm

Ford, Vicki. *Overcoming Sexual Problems*, 2nd edition. London: Robinson. 2017.

https://www.citizensinformation.ie/en/justice/law_enforcement/monitoring_sex_offenders_in_ireland.html

https://www.harleytherapy.co.uk/sexual-problems-help-guide.htmht   https://www.harleytherapy.co.uk/sexual-problems-help-guide.htmtps://www.harl

Losing count of the calories

Starting slowly, skip a meal here, cut a bit out there. This suits my student budget. There is no harm in eating less, loads of people skip breakfast. I hear your compliments, I revel in them, repeating them in my head when I think of food. I step on the scale once a week, the thrill of losing weight rushing through me, propelling me through my day. I could accomplish anything. It faded. I am once again a struggling student. Why am I struggling? More weight lost. Euphoria. Power, control and invincibility. Losing weight is healthy. I am eating enough; I wish you would butt out and leave me to enjoy this newfound magic.

More weight lost. Daily weighing. Cutting this down, skipping that. Could I replace this with something lighter? One gym class. Happiness. Lightness. Two, three, four, five, six classes. Run, cycle, run, cycle, walk everywhere, counting steps, calories, weight lost.

More weight loss. Joy. Sadness. Why am I sad? I need to lose more; I need to feel good enough. Why don't I set a target? Counting, calories, days, laxatives, gym classes, steps, weight loss, meals skipped, money saved.

Target reached. I step off the scales. Euphoria. I can do anything. This is my body now. I decide what I do with my body. I am in control. I put the scales away, and feel sadness, empty, ugly and fat. I need to lose more now. New target. Counting, steps, laxatives, calories, gym classes, runs, meals skipped, meals eaten, social activities missed, university essays piling up.

Target reached. Nothing. Missed calls, missed lectures, missed meals, missed weekends home. New target. Counting, steps, calories, laxatives, purging, runs, gym classes, meals eaten, meals skipped, weight lost, lies told. Nothing. Weight not moving. Fear, panic, shame, anger. Three times daily weighing just to show myself how weak and useless I am. Counting, missed calls, missed texts, panic attacks, laxatives, purging, diet pills, calories, gym classes, runs, walks, steps, meals eaten, meals skipped, social activities missed, relationships ending, lectures missed, deadlines missed, essays piling up, lies told, minutes and seconds till I can eat again.

Target reached. Nothing else matters now. This is my life, my body. Sadness, feeling fat, cannot sleep. I need a new target. I could try a liquid diet. I am not hungry; hunger is for the weak. Food is an addiction, and we are eating too much. Everyone is lying to me. I am not thin; I am not sick. I am in control, I am strong. I walk through the shop, eyeing up the food, smug. I am more powerful than you, I do not need you. I am not stupid like everyone else. I am not addicted to food. I am strong, I am strong. I am strong.

Bathroom floor, tears, dizziness, tiredness, sore throat, weakness, thoughts about all the food, enjoying the thoughts of food. Imagining the taste, the texture, the temperature. Guilt, I am strong. I do not need food. I am powerful. I am in control. Counting, steps, calories, runs, gym classes, weight lost, missed calls, missed lectures, lies told, missed meals, friends lost, essays piling up, time spent in bed, time spent on the bathroom floor, nights without sleep, days missed. Sadness, guilt. I am drinking too many liquids. Fasting, hours counting down on the app on my phone, I can fast longer than anyone on this app. I am strong.

I am scared. I am not thin enough. Guilt for sleeping when I could be running. Guilt for doing badly at university. Loneliness. Emptiness, sadness, weakness. Counting, steps, calories, laxatives, diet pills, purging, runs, gym classes, lectures missed, friends lost, essays piling up, time spent on the bathroom floor, nights without sleep, weight lost. Then weakness, stomach pain, fatigue, dizziness. Counting, calories, doctor visits, stomach tablets, diet pills, laxatives, runs, gym classes, wait, I cannot remember, what am I supposed to be counting?

Days lost, days in bed, hours slept. Cannot concentrate, cannot remember. Loneliness, powerlessness, fear. Dead. Trapped. Lost. Alone. Fear. Panic attacks. Tears. Powerlessness. Guilt. Stomach pain. Dizziness. Cold. Did I miss a period? I cannot remember.

Loneliness, hopelessness, powerlessness. Weight lost. Targets reached. New batteries for the weighing scales. Guilt. Chewing food for taste, spitting it back out for happiness. Isolation. Fear. I think I need help.

Hello, counselling service, please leave your name, number and details and we will get back to you. Shame, embarrassment. I muttered my name; I think I am struggling to eat a little. I forget to add my number. Hello, counselling service, I repeat and apologise, I add my number.

Waiting. Fear. Shame. Embarrassment. Phone rings. Appointment booked. Guilt, I am not sick enough to get help. I will waste their time.

You come out and smile. I count the steps it would take for me to run. I am too tired; I cannot fight any more. I follow you. You tell me it's OK, you can see how much I am struggling. I stand and face the scales, ashamed, I am too fat, and you will see now too just how fat and useless I am. We talk, I am ashamed, I feel guilty. You ask me to eat one piece of chicken a day for the week. I leave, I cry, I can't do it, your words play in my head, you will die, you're sick, you need food, you will collapse if you keep going, your degree is at risk. You have anorexia.

13

Mind and Body Disorders

Somatoform disorders are psychiatric ones that manifest themselves through physical symptoms. What this means is the physical symptoms the person describes are related to psychological factors instead of a medical cause. These are the most difficult psychiatric conditions to explain to the public.

Up to the modern era, and even into the 20th century, many people believed that the mind and the body were separate and distinct entities. The 16th-century French philosopher René Descartes (of 'I think therefore I am' fame) expressed this in his philosophy of 'dualism', according to which the mind 'controls' the body as if it is a 'ghost in the machine'. This was the perspective that medicine adhered to for centuries. In the course of the 20th century it became apparent that this theory is false, and that there is in fact significant overlap between mind and body. This change in perspective has been assisted by developments in neuroscience, and by the impact this perspective has had on the treatment initiatives for what were hitherto regarded as disorders solely of the mind, such as schizophrenia.

This chapter will address three aspects of the mind-body link:

- Physical symptoms in psychiatric disorders
- Psychological reactions to physical illness
- Physical symptoms that are medically unexplained (medically unexplained symptoms, or MUS)

The term 'psychosomatic' is a well recognised one among the general public. It refers to a group of medical conditions that are made worse by underlying mental health issues. These include conditions like hypertension, eczema, stomach ulcers etc., although these connections are difficult to prove. The term is also used to describe physical symptoms that are caused by mental health factors. These are discussed below (p.231f.), but the term psychosomatic will not be used – instead the term 'somatoform' will be preferred.

COMMON PHYSICAL SYMPTOMS IN PSYCHIATRIC DISORDERS

Depressive illness (see Chapter 7), adjustment disorders (see Chapter 4), and anxiety disorder disorders (see Chapter 5) are very common in the general population. They are often overshadowed by prominent physical symptoms. For example, sleep disturbance, aches and pains, palpitations, sleep changes and reduced appetite with significant weight loss are common features of depressive illness in particular. Palpitations, difficulty breathing, and dizziness accompanied by sense of impending death are described in those experiencing panic attacks. These symptoms may lead to a slew of physical investigations to rule out heart disease, arthritis, gastrointestinal disorders, atrial fibrillation, thyroid disease and so on. Withdrawal from alcohol can cause sweating, high blood pressure and palpitations. The person experiencing these symptoms may mistakenly think they have a heart condition unless questions are asked about alcohol use.

Your doctor will quite rightly investigate such symptoms; indeed, so close is the overlap that it is important to rule out a serious physical illness as the cause of the symptoms. Likewise, it is judicious to cease reasonable tests for these when the findings are negative. In addition, considering a physical illness as the cause has to be done in the context of a detailed history of psychological symptoms and careful annotation of the timeline of physical symptoms alongside the emotional symptoms.

Case Vignette

Mrs A, aged 75, lost her husband about five months before referral to a psychiatrist. She had lost 10kg in weight and also had appetite loss, nausea, discomfort on eating, and loss of interest and taste for food. She was tired and weak and had trouble staying asleep. She felt sad and lonely. She attributed her sleep problems to worry about her physical state. Gastrointestinal investigations were normal. Her GP advised her that she might be still grieving for the loss of her husband. When seen she described having no difficulty crying for her loss but feeling lonely as the couple had had a very good companionship. They married late in life and had no children. She had lost interest in visiting her siblings and her late husband's family. She was able to visit the grave. Numerous physical investigations on the gastrointestinal tract and related blood tests were also normal.

Once it was established that this lady did not have any physical explanation for her symptoms, it was reasonable, in the context of a recent bereavement, to consider a depressive illness as the likely diagnosis. Bereavement counselling might be considered later in the course of her treatment but in the first instance, due to her typical biological symptoms of a depressive episode, including significant weight loss, she was commenced on an antidepressant and responded very rapidly. Bereavement counselling will be indicated if she has trouble coming to terms with the loss of her husband, although loneliness would be regarded as understandable. Bereavement therapy for normal grief is likely to prolong grief and is therefore not indicated.

Comment:
This lady had serious physical symptoms that might lead to consideration of a physical illness. Other conditions also need to be explored when specific symptoms are present.
The obvious conclusion is that when reasonable tests have excluded a physical illness as the explanation, consider a psychiatric disorder as a likely alternative.

Note: This is not a real case, but it describes a typical scenario.

PSYCHOLOGICAL REACTIONS TO PHYSICAL ILLNESS

Psychiatric illnesses, then, can have physical symptoms. But it goes the other way too: Psychiatric symptoms occur in many physical illnesses as an inherent part of the physical condition. Viral infections can cause lethargy and depressed mood, and thyroid disease can cause anxiety or depressive symptoms as well as physical symptoms. Those who are diabetic and who suffer hypoglycaemic episodes (i.e. bouts of low blood sugar) can present with acute psychotic symptoms and become agitated, paranoid or confused. Certain cancers cause low mood, believed to be more than just the understandable sadness of having a life-threatening illness. In some cases depressed mood is present before the cancer is even diagnosed. It is believed that changes in the release of cortisol and melatonin from parts of the brain and the impact of depression on the immune system is responsible (Spiegel and Gleese-David, 2003).

Physical illnesses can also have *indirect* psychiatric conditions. For instance, low mood can be a response to a physical illness simply because the illness is debilitating or has a high mortality. In that case, the emotional response is not an *inherent* part of that illness, but the person's response to it. Distinguishing what is a normal emotional response to a serious illness, and what is excessive and in need of an intervention, can be challenging, and is fraught with the danger of over-diagnosis of psychiatric disorder (see Chapter 4). A person with a life-threatening illness such as cancer may feel low in mood and stressed, and because of worry may have difficulty sleeping or focusing on anything other than their illness, but in the face of such a terrible looming possibility, is this not an appropriate response? Deciding when treatment with antidepressants is needed, rather than just a listening ear and support, is difficult and a matter for careful consideration. In most cases talking therapies are preferred by people going through such a difficult time in their life. A study found that adjustment disorder/stress (see Chapter 4) was more slightly common than depressive illness in those with cancer (Mitchell et al., 2011), confirming the need for talk therapy slightly more than medication. Even when the response to a cancer or similar diagnosis is considered understandable and proportionate, and not a psychiatric condition, there is still a place for listening, explaining and answering questions, and that is why good medical services also provide specially trained counsellors, particularly for those who do not have the support that they need from family or the space to vent their fears and frustrations regarding their diagnosis and treatment.

MEDICALLY UNEXPLAINED SYMPTOMS (MUS) OR SOMATOFORM DISORDERS

Somatoform disorders are the most difficult group of conditions to grasp and to manage clinically. Somatoform disorders are now called somatic symptom disorders in the US text that describes these conditions (DSM-5). In the WHO documents, used throughout Europe, the terminology is set to change in 2022 in ICD-11. Somatoform disorders will be called disorders of bodily distress or bodily experience. The names of other conditions such as hypochondriasis are also changing to health anxiety.

Why is the terminology in this area of psychiatry so fluid? It is indicative either of the limited understanding we have of these conditions or of the fact that we are gaining more knowledge about how they relate to other conditions in psychiatry.

The definition of somatoform disorders is that they consist of physical symptoms that suggest illness or injury but for which no adequate medical explanation exists, and they are not attributable to another psychiatric disorder. Some that were regarded as somatoform, are now recognised as more closely related to anxiety or to OCD. Nevertheless, for simplicity they are described below.

Somatoforms and similar conditions

- **Somatic symptom disorder/somatisation disorder/bodily distress disorder:** A condition in which someone has physical symptoms without any medical cause. These may be in multiple systems: for instance, the person may have symptoms in both the digestive (e.g. gastrointestinal with abdominal pain), neurological and muscular systems (e.g. pins and needles and pain in the muscles of the legs), or many other combinations. These symptoms are persistent, but there is no medical condition that can explain the combination.

- **Conversion disorder:** This is a condition in which the person has a physical function impairment of sudden onset – for instance, blindness, numbness, fits or some other condition of the nervous system – that cannot be medically explained. These people are not 'making up' their symptoms (they are not malingering), nor are they intentionally injuring themselves to become a patient (factitious disorder; see p.232). These symptoms usually begin after a major trauma and are most likely a subconscious attempt to resolve an inner emotional conflict. Most recover after a few days or weeks if given talking therapy and physiotherapy.

- **Dissociation:** This occurs when the person feels cut off from themselves and/or the world around them. They may have amnesia, they may forget who they are or wander away from home in a lost state. Depersonalisation and derealisation (see Chapter 5) are milder manifestations of dissociation. The most stark manifestation, though, is dissociative identity disorder (DID), also called 'multiple personality disorder'. For all the representation DID has had in popular culture – where it is often erroneously conflated with 'schizophrenia,' which is in fact an entirely different condition (see Chapter 8) – there is scepticism and debate among psychiatrists as to its existence. Conversion and dissociation were formerly referred to as hysteria, after Freud gave these states this name.

- **Factitious disorder:** This consists of self-induced injuries or symptoms which the patient uses to meet a psychological need, usually for care. For instance, the person will put a substance in their urine to make it seem as if they are passing blood, or they will pick open a wound so as to infect it, leading to hospitalisation. The motivation is to seek care and attention. Factitious disorder differs from malingering, which is not a psychiatric illness, and refers to a person who exaggerates or fabricates symptoms to achieve an external goal, e.g. compensation from an accident, deferral of a trial in court.

- **Pain disorder:** In this disorder, a person has pain despite the absence of any physical or other evidence of a cause. Sometimes there is initially a physical cause, but the pain persists long after the cause subsides. For instance, a strain injury might cause legitimate pain, but the person may find that even after the injury has healed, the pain continues. Talking about it and continuing the investigations can prolong it. This occurs without any deliberate exaggeration. When it is knowingly exaggerated for gain, e.g. after an accident, it is called malingering. Distinguishing true pain disorder from malingering can be very difficult.

- **Hypochondriasis/health anxiety:** These are simply two names for a single condition. The definition is worrying to excess that a

> serious illness will occur. Commonly there are no physical symptoms present or, if they do occur, they are an over-sensitivity to and misinterpretation of normal bodily sensations.
>
> • **Bodily integrity dysphoria:** This is a very rare and under-researched condition in which an individual has a discomfort with being able-bodied or has a desire to be disabled by amputation or being rendered deaf, blind etc. Some are sexually aroused by such thoughts. Surgery in such cases raises huge ethical questions. It is a very controversial condition.

The reaction of the person to unexplained symptoms may vary greatly, from those who are stoic and accept the fact that no physical cause has been found, to those who constantly seek out different doctors and further investigations. Attitudes vary in the medical profession, from doctors who disbelieve the person and accuse them of making up the symptoms, to those who are sympathetic and are able to offer an explanation in psychological terms that link the physical to the psychological. Those with unexplained symptoms experience low mood, anxiety and general distress at the presence of the symptoms, as well as at the failure to find a physical cause.

CHRONIC FATIGUE SYNDROME/MYALGIC ENCEPHALOMYELITIS

The conundrum of the physical/psychological divide is most clearly shown in the debate about chronic fatigue syndrome (otherwise known as myalgic encephalomyelitis) (CFS/ME). This was formerly known by the derogatory term 'yuppie flu' when it first emerged in the 1980s. Before that, almost two centuries ago, the term 'neurasthenia' was used to describe a similar condition, and interest in it was renewed when the concept was reintroduced by George Miller Beard in 1869. It continued to be used in psychiatry until the 1980s, when the new terminology emerged.

That CFS/ME has two names is a reflection of the fact that there are two theories about the condition's origin: one indicating a physical origin (ME), the other a psychological one (CFS).

The symptoms often begin after a flu-like illness. Glands may be swollen. The key feature is significant tiredness, which, along with muscle weakness and pain, may make exercise very difficult. At times the tiredness is so profound that it renders the person bed-bound. Raised blood pressure and a thumping heart (palpitations) are also common symptoms. Thought processes and concentration may be impaired.

The treatments that are offered reflect the differences in the perceived causation, with some focusing on triggering stressors, on cognitive therapy along with graded exercises, and others focusing on anti-viral treatments, immuno-suppressants and symptomatic treatment of headaches, insomnia and other symptoms. If the condition is psychological in nature, then it is likely triggered by stressors and the symptoms are likely maintained by psychosocial factors; if, however, the condition is primarily physical, biological processes are responsible.

There are no diagnostic tests for CFS/ME, and no pathologies have been identified in the tissues or organs involved in those suffering from it. Moreover, a diagnosis can take a long time because it cannot be made until physical causes of the key symptoms have first been ruled out. In terms of expected outcome of those diagnosed with it, some improve, others run a 'fluctuating course' in which things cycle between good and bad periods over many months, and around 25% remain seriously incapacitated, unable to work or socialise. The impact on finances and on relationships can be very serious.

The debates on the nature of this condition often focus on the stigmatising effect of a psychiatric diagnosis, on the absence of biological markers, and on the failure to show benefits from specific psychiatric interventions. The debate continues.

 ## WHAT YOU CAN DO FOR YOURSELF AND WHAT OTHERS CAN DO FOR YOU

- If somebody has unexplained medical symptoms that have been investigated do not encourage further investigations.
- Do not tell the person that their physical complaints are all in their mind.
- Find a cognitive therapist who understands health anxiety and somatoform disorders.
- Offer support without engaging in detailed conversation about their symptoms.
- Encourage those with CFS/ME to read self-help guides.

BIBLIOGRAPHY

Mitchell, A., Chan, M., Bhatti, H. et al. 'Prevalence of depression, anxiety, and adjustment disorder in oncological, haematological and palliative-care settings: a meta-analysis of 94 interview-based studies'. *Lancet Oncol.* 2011; 12 (2): 160–74.

Spiegel, David and Giese-Davis, Janine. 'Depression and cancer: mechanisms and disease progression'. *Biological Psychiatry.* 54, 3. 269–82. 2003.

USEFUL RESOURCES

Burgess, Mary, with Chalder, Trudie. *Overcoming Chronic Fatigue.* London: Robinson. 2009.

Hogan, Brenda. *An Introduction to Coping with Health Anxiety.* London: Robinson. 2017.

O'Sullivan, Suzanne. *It's all in Your Head: Stories from the Frontline of Psychosomatic Illness.* New York, NY: Vintage. 2016.

Sharp, Michael and Campling, Frankie. *Chronic Fatigue Syndrome: The Facts.* Oxford: Oxford University Press. 2000.

https://www.rcpsych.ac.uk/mental-health/problems-disorders/medically-unexplained-symptoms

NICE draft Guidelines updated: Diagnosis and Management CFS/ME 2020.

The Three Faces of Eve. 1957 (a movie about DID).

Schreiber, Flora Rheya. *Sybil.* 1973 (a novel about DID).

14

Legal and Ethical Issues in Psychiatry

Psychiatry is the only medical specialty that can detain and treat certain people against their will. It is a unique power, but also a heavy responsibility: if used inappropriately, it would be a gross breach of human rights. In contrast, the ethics of confidentiality apply to *all* medical specialties. This chapter deals with compulsory detention and treatment, and the related issues of capacity to make decisions about various aspects of one's life, and confidentiality in relation to mental health.

COMPULSORY DETENTION UNDER THE MENTAL HEALTH ACT 2001

The compulsory treatment of patients was revamped with the enactment of The Mental Health Act in 2001. Prior to this, people had to 'sign themselves in' to hospital. This was based on the Mental Treatment Act 1945. The new legislation took a different a approach: now, people can be admitted to hospital without having to sign themselves in. If a person requires inpatient treatment but refuses it, then the Mental Health Act 2001 can, under certain circumstances, be used to detain the person compulsorily.

Ireland's involuntary admission rate of 46.7 people per 100,000 is low by international standards; 12% of admissions annually are compulsory, and the most common diagnosis in those compulsorily admitted is schizophrenia, followed by mania and depressive disorders (Kelly, 2017).

Compulsorily admitting someone to hospital is a serious infringement of their liberty, so the grounds under which it can happen are specified very precisely. In summary, a person can be compulsorily admitted to hospital if:

(a) because of the illness, disability or dementia, there is a serious likelihood that they will cause immediate and serious harm to themselves or others,

and/or

(b) (i) their judgement is so impaired that failure to admit them would be likely to lead to serious deterioration in this condition and would prevent the use of treatment that could only be given by such admission, and (ii) the detention and treatment of the person would be likely to benefit or alleviate the condition of that person to a material extent (Mental Health Act 2001).

Only one of (a) or (b) above is required, though both can be present.

THE PROCESS OF COMPULSORY ADMISSION:

A number of steps have to be followed when a compulsory admission is required. The first is that an application is made for the admission of the person to a psychiatric unit. This has to be on the list of 'approved centres' recognised by the Mental Health Commission, the statutory body that oversees psychiatric facilities in Ireland.

The forms for this process are available from GP surgeries, from a member of the mental health team or from the Mental Health Commission or its website. The completion of this form does not require any knowledge of psychiatry and can be filled out by anyone: it is a layperson's account of the behaviour or symptoms causing concern.

The application

The application is usually made through the GP, but the form can also be given directly by the applicant to the approved centre. The applicant must have seen the person within 48 hours of writing the application; they may be a spouse, a civil partner, a relative, a member of An Garda Síochána, an 'authorised officer' or a member of the public. An authorised officer is a member of the health service who is specifically designated the task of making these applications, if nobody else is available or willing to do so. They can be reached through the community mental health team. If a relative does not wish to make the application, perhaps through fear or from not wanting to upset their relationship with the ill person, the authorised officer may do so instead. Certain people are prohibited from doing so, including a spouse from whom the person is separated or against whom an order has been made under the Domestic Violence Act 2018, a doctor who provides a GP service to the approved centre, or those under the age of 18

If the Gardaí are called, they will either take the person to the emergency department of the hospital where the approved centre is located or into Garda custody, and the admission process will commence there. Note that the Gardaí can be involved in an involuntary admission only if ground (a) above is cited, i.e. if the person presents a danger of serious and immediate harm to themselves or others.

The recommendation

This second step involves a registered medical practitioner who does not work at the approved centre completing the recommendation form. This is usually a GP, although it may sometimes be a doctor in the emergency department of the hospital to which the patient has been taken. If the person is in Garda custody, the Gardaí may take the person to the emergency department or they may call a GP to the Garda station. The doctor is not obliged to sign the admission form, and will not do so if of the opinion that the person does not meet the criteria for compulsory admission. These forms are then sent to the approved centre. If the patient has been seen at home by the doctor making the recommendation but still refuses to come to hospital, the consultant psychiatrist who will receive the patient in hospital is obliged to arrange for an assisted admission. This is done with specially trained personnel who will go to the person's house and take them to the named psychiatric facility.

The admission order

When the patient arrives at the approved centre, they must be seen by the consultant psychiatrist, who decides whether they meet the criteria for compulsory admission detailed above. The doctor will not complete the form if they do not believe that the criteria are met. If they do complete the admission order, though, the initial authorisation is for a period of 21 days. Once the patient has been certified, the Mental Health Commission is notified and the process of an independent health tribunal to review the order commences immediately. The tribunal must hold its hearing within 21 days of the signing of the order.

At any time between making the committal order and the hearing by the tribunal, the order may be revoked by the consultant. This often happens and, when it does, it is almost always either because the patient has improved to the extent that they no longer need to be compulsorily detained, or because they are willing to remain as a voluntary patient.

The mental health tribunal

This tribunal conducts the hearing in the unit to which the patient has been admitted. It consists of a lawyer, a psychiatrist and a layperson trained for this type of hearing through the Mental Health Commission. It hears oral evidence from the psychiatrist under whose care the patient has been admitted. The patient may give evidence if they wish and they are provided with their own solicitor to whom they give instructions. In advance of the hearing, an independent psychiatrist will also assess the patient. The hearings are non-adversarial and are conducted with the patient's best interests in mind.

If the patient no longer meets the criteria for detention because their condition has improved, or if there was some procedural irregularity such as forms being completed incorrectly, the tribunal will revoke the admission order. If the tribunal affirms the order and it remains in place, the person must remain in hospital. The patient can appeal the decision of the tribunal to the Circuit Court if they wish, and in this event a court hearing will follow.

The renewal order

If, following the mental health tribunal, the person remains in hospital detained under the Mental Health Act, a renewal order is signed. A second tribunal is held no later than three months after the signing of the order. The patient continues to have the services of a solicitor.

Other considerations

If the person is admitted *voluntarily* to hospital, and they wish to leave against medical advice, they are free to do so. However, if there are concerns that they are not well enough to leave and meet the criteria for compulsory detention outlined above, the process of certification can be initiated. In this instance, an independent psychiatrist will be called to decide on the appropriateness of this decision before the treating psychiatrist makes the final order. The process of holding a tribunal, as described above, will then commence.

The mental health legislation itself cannot force *physically* ill people to have treatment against their will in *any* circumstances. For example, a patient with cancer who is refusing treatment for this, but is not able to give full and free consent, perhaps because of confusion, cannot be detained under the Mental Health Act and given treatment. A court order would be required to treat them for cancer against their wishes and this would require an assessment of their capacity.

It is clear from the above that the public belief in somebody 'being signed into hospital' is erroneous and simplistic. Instead, it is a careful and multi-stage process that has many protections for the patient, from second opinions to free legal representation. Moreover, the idea of a person 'signing' themselves out of hospital is an outmoded one also, since patients are almost always *voluntarily* admitted and can, except in very specific circumstances, leave voluntarily too.

The Mental Health Act 2001 is available online by simply inserting 'Mental Health Act Ireland 2001' into your browser, or by contacting Citizens Information for further ideatils.

DETENTION UNDER THE CRIMINAL LAW INSANITY ACT 2006

The Criminal Law Insanity Act 2006 applies to those charged with a criminal offence who are suffering from a psychiatric disorder. This law is only relevant to those charged with a crime who have a *serious* mental health disorder. The definition of 'mental disorder' excludes intoxication and personality disorder. Details of this legislation are available online simply by inserting 'Criminal Law Insanity Act 2006' into your browser.

The act comes into play in advance of the trial for an offence when the person's *fitness to be tried* is questioned. Being fit to be tried means that the person must be able to follow the trial, must remember what is said, must be able to instruct the legal team, must understand what a plea of 'guilty' means, and must also understand the role of the judge and jury. Someone with a learning disability or a serious mental illness may not understand some of these elements, and would therefore be found unfit to be tried. They would be re-assessed after a period of treatment.

Even if the defendant is fit to be tried, they may be 'not guilty by reason of insanity', or claim diminished responsibility. In the former case, the person may plead that they are not guilty of the crime with which they have been charged by reason of insanity, even if they have committed the offence. A person taking the life of another under instruction from voices commanding them to do so might be an example of where this plea is used. In the latter case, the defendant may plead diminished responsibility. On this defence, the defendant would still be deemed responsible for their actions, but the charge would be reduced, for instance from murder to manslaughter.

The criteria for testing fitness to be tried, not guilty by reason of insanity, or diminished responsibility are laid out in the act itself. Further details of this are also available from Citizens Information. Whether a defendant meets any of these criteria is obviously a matter of some importance, and if any are claimed, this requires thorough assessment by experts familiar with this type of assessment, usually but not always, forensic psychiatrists.

Notwithstanding the existence of the Criminal Law Insanity Act, this should not be used to assume that there is an absolute link between severe mental illness and violent crime. Most people with mental health problems do not engage in significant criminal behaviour and most violent crimes are not committed by the mentally ill. However, a small group of patients with severe mental illness have an increased risk of perpetrating violent crime if untreated (Mullen, 2009). The presence of severe mental illness with substance misuse is a major risk factor for violence in schizophrenia. Thus, reducing substance misuse and ensuring continuing adherence to treatment is crucial but difficult to ensure.

WHAT IS CAPACITY?

'Capacity' is defined in psychiatric circles as the ability to make an informed decision about some aspect of one's life. In law, this is defined broadly enough that almost everyone has capacity. However, if there is doubt about a person's ability to make a particular decision for themselves, such as a healthcare decision, a *capacity assessment* is required. When such an assessment is required, the person's solicitor is informed of the concern.

If the person is feared to lack capacity in relation to their financial affairs, consideration will be given to making them a ward of court. This usually arises when a person has severe dementia or brain damage following an accident or due to a learning disability. In this instance two medical practitioners have to provide an opinion and the Office of Wards of Court will also send an independent doctor to evaluate the person. The court will then make a decision based on the evidence presented by the doctors and any other relevant witnesses. They will be examined and cross-examined on their findings as in any court hearing.

A person can have capacity without making a good, wise or 'correct' decision. All that is required is that the person can go through a process of understanding the issue in question and can weigh up alternatives.

Case Vignette

Mr A, a 65-year-old single man, was a patient on a surgical ward and was due to have surgery for cancer of the bowel. He refused surgery, saying he would rather die than have this. He said chemotherapy should be tried first. He had in the past been treated for a depressive illness, the last time eight years ago. The surgeon wanted to check if this man had the capacity to make this decision. He said he had informed Mr A that chemotherapy would not of itself help and that surgery was essential to save his life.

Comment:
The starting point would be to evaluate whether Mr A now had a recurrence of his depressive illness, leading him to want to die or causing an excessive fear of the surgery. If his concentration is impaired he may not have fully understood the information he was given about the procedure. Following an interview with Mr A and with his next of

kin, his sister, and his GP, there was no evidence that he was now suffering with depression. He was aware that without surgery the prognosis was poor and that if he had surgery he could go for convalescence to a nursing home for a period. He repeatedly said that he would not have surgery and that he had no fear of death. He said surgery would not necessarily cure his cancer as it could come back again. He said he would wish to go to a hospice once he was discharged from hospital.

Mr A had capacity, even though he was making a poor decision in respect of his treatment. He could understand the information he was given and relay it to the interviewer. He gave reasons for making his decision, despite the information he had about prognosis. He was aware of his options post-operatively and rejected them. He cannot be compelled to have surgery. A prudent course would be to provide further information about convalescence and try gentle persuasion by his family. He may change his mind. His decision must be respected. This is an example of a person making a poor decision but having capacity.

Note: This is not a true case but is the type of situation that often arises in hospitals.

CAN CAPACITY BE REGAINED?

Capacity can sometimes be regained if there is a treatment for the condition causing the lack of capacity. Thus the capacity assessment is only valid at the time when the assessment is made and in respect of the specific issue that has been tested. Thus, a person planning on making a will may lack capacity when first tested, but regain it a few months later after treatment. Likewise, capacity in one area, e.g. making a will, does not mean that the person has capacity in another area, e.g. making health decisions. Each has to be evaluated separately.

When there is no treatment to help a person regain capacity, such as when they have dementia, a learning disability or a brain injury, the solution is to make them a ward of court. The court will appoint a committee to act on behalf of the ward and make the assets available for the benefit of the ward. The committee will control their financial and other assets, and make decisions concerning travel, health and marriage on behalf of the court. For these reasons wardship is not lightly entered into.

HOW TO ASSESS CAPACITY

A capacity assessment takes the form of an interview in which various questions are asked of the person being assessed.

The basic principles of capacity assessment are summarised below.

Elements of capacity assessment

The person must be:

- aware of the issue that is being examined, e.g. financial or health decisions;

- able to understand the questions;

- able to retain the information;

- able to weight up the options, such as risks/benefits/alternatives to the course of action chosen;

- able to remember their decisions.

Once the person's ability to hear and comprehend language and re-member information is established, the next part of the interview is di-rected to ensuring that they understand what issue is being examined, e.g. the ability to manage their financial affairs. This is followed by ques-tions specific to the area under consideration.

In an assessment of a person's ability to manage their financial af-fairs, they must be able to tell the assessor the value of their estate, the name of their bank, and the basic details of their bank accounts. They must know how to withdraw money from their accounts and have information on who else knows about their accounts, and how that person came to have that knowledge. Questions about the value of common everyday items and what the person's approximate spending is over any given period will be very useful for assessing their day-to-day management of their affairs. Basic addition and subtraction will provide information on their safety with money. Some may have safe-guards in place, such as using a calculator in shops. If they have money for investing they should be able to weigh up the pros and cons of a particular investment being proposed. The potential for exploitation by others is also relevant and the person's ability to protect themselves from this must be considered.

The questions will be slightly different for somebody wanting to make a will. In this instance they must be aware of the size of their estate and how much it is worth. They must have the name of the person to whom they will bequeath their property, other people or organisations who could benefit and the reasons for choosing these. The person must be able to recall discussions with their solicitor. They must be able to explain why they have chosen a particular person or organisation for the inheritance. The person must be shown to be free from coercion regarding their decision. Those who lack capacity are vulnerable to coercion, referred to as 'undue influence'. They may also be asked to do some basic addition and subtraction to help establish if they are able to manage money.

For any area being assessed, it is not enough for the person passively to agree with everything the assessor asks. The individual must be able to demonstrate an *active* ability to consider the matters in hand and to weigh up risks and benefits, when these apply.

Capacity can be assessed in a number of areas, listed below.

Areas of capacity assessment

- Capacity to manage one's financial or business affairs
- Fitness to be tried for a criminal offence
- Testamentary capacity (fitness to make a will)
- Capacity to marry
- Capacity to consent to a specific treatment
- Capacity to consent to release of information, e.g. to relatives when ill (and see Confidentiality, p.248)

Among psychiatric inpatients admitted voluntarily, around 30% lack capacity to make treatment decisions, and this rises to 89% among involuntary patients (Owens, 2008).

THE ASSISTED DECISION-MAKING (CAPACITY) ACT 2015

Making a person a ward of court is a serious decision: it risks being draconian since it robs the person of autonomy to a significant degree. Making the decision is complicated by 'tough cases' that fall on the boundaries of the definition of 'capacity'. There are situations where an individual has not lost *all* capacity, and who is largely able to manage their affairs with some independent assistance. The view among doctors involved in such cases was that a less rigid approach was required, and new legislation called the Assisted Decision-Making (Capacity) Act 2015 was signed into law in December 2015. As yet, though, it has not become operational and the Lunacy Regulation Act 1871 continues to be used.

The 2015 Act recognises that three levels of decision-making are required, depending on the degree of incapacity identified. All are subject to various restrictions under the act.

Levels of decision-making in the Assisted Decision-Making (Capacity) Act 2015.

- **Decision-making assistant** – Their role is similar to what happens in day-to-day life where we seek advice from others. The assistant has no decision-making responsibility.

- **Co-decision maker** – This person makes the decision jointly with the impaired person, and this is formally registered.

- **Substitute decision-maker** – This person makes the decision *for* the person, having first attempted to establish their will and preference.

Unlike the legislation in England and Wales, Northern Ireland, and Scotland, where the 'best interests' of the person is an overarching principle, in the Irish act the focus is on facilitating autonomy and avoiding paternalism. There is also a legitimate concern that incorporating 'best interests' into the Irish act could cause it to conflict with the Constitution.

The act has two other important elements. The first is the power for someone who currently has capacity to nominate somebody to act on their behalf should they lose it, for example if they develop dementia. This is known as enduring power of attorney. This would ordinarily also be discussed with a solicitor. The application has to be registered with the Decision Support Service, and it activates once the solicitor becomes aware that the donor lacks capacity, should that ever come to pass. Thereafter annual reports must be provided by the solicitor to the Decision Support Service, indicating that the person continues to lack capacity.

The second element in the act is specifically focused on healthcare. It deals with the right to make decisions about future care during a period of well-being. This is known colloquially as a 'living will', or an advance-healthcare directive (AHC). It is believed that these give people greater autonomy, with less need for coercion, and will improve the relationship between healthcare professionals and the patient during a period of hos-pitalisation. The AHC gives an indication of the treatment one wishes to receive or refuse should one become ill in the future and lackcapacity. For example, a person with bipolar disorder who is currently well might specify that during a future episode of illness they do not wish to receive certain medications or treatments, such as ECT. Although the request for a specific treatment is not legally binding, it has to be taken into consideration.

Nobody yet knows when the 2015 act will become operational.

CONFIDENTIALITY

Confidentiality is the cornerstone of the doctor-patient relationship. It means that anything disclosed to a doctor during a consultation cannot be divulged to anyone else without that person's consent. This is the case even for illegal or immoral activities. So, if you tell your doctor that you have abused cocaine or have been unfaithful to your partner, for instance, this disclosure stays between you and your doctor. This gives you the security of knowing that your trust will not be betrayed. This applies to doctors in *all* specialties, be it general practice, psychiatry or anything else. However, the ethics of confidentiality is *not absolute*, and there are situations in which confidentiality can and, even must, be broken. These will be discussed below

Implicit and explicit permission

Permission to disclose information may be *implicit* or *explicit*. *Implicit* permission is an assumption that, without discussion, health-related in-formation will be passed on to a third party. A typical example is when your GP refers you to a specialist. They will include relevant information about your condition to assist that specialist without specifically obtain-ing your permission. However, information *not* pertinent to the reasons for your referral will obviously not be divulged, and the GP has no legal right to disclose this information. By contrast, *explicit* permission re-quires either verbal or written permission for disclosure.

If, for instance, a GP referred you to a gastroenterologist for a suspect-ed stomach ulcer, they would not need explicit permission to detail your symptoms, including a history of alcohol abuse and relevant family history of having ulcers, since both are relevant to your condition. This would be an example of implicit permission. If more peripheral information were to be provided, e.g. that in the past you were charged with fraud, your GP would need to obtain explicit permission from you. The information dis-closed to a fellow professional should be relevant and proportionate to the requirements of the specialist. For example, referral from a GP to a surgeon for treatment of an ulcer would require different information from that given to a psychiatrist, who would normally be provided with details of the person's social, personal and past psychiatric history.

For the release of information to non-medical bodies, explicit written permission is always required. This would include requests from banks, insurance companies and housing authorities. The information provided must be very specific and focus only on the stated purpose for which it is requested. For example, if you are applying for a mortgage, you will be asked about prior illnesses, including those of a psychiatric nature. This may result in the lender requesting a report on your condition from the treating psychiatrist. This request may stem from concerns about long-term unemployment due to illness and inability to make repayments. An insurer underwriting the mortgage might inquire about suicide risk. In responding to these requests, a psychiatrist can disclose the person's psychiatric history *only if the person explicitly grants them permission to do so*, since these are non-medical agencies. In almost all instances that I have dealt with, written permission from the patient for the release of information was included in the request to me.

Breaking confidentiality

In certain circumstances confidentiality may be broken against the patient's wishes. These circumstances are divided into four categories, as follows:

1. **When there is a danger to the patient themselves:** This arises, for example, if a person divulges suicidal thoughts and plans, and if

their psychiatrist thinks that there is a credible and immediate risk of them acting on these thoughts and plans. The patient may request that their next of kin not be informed. However, in a high-risk situation such as this, the psychiatrist must inform their next of kin (or another person close to the patient). This is in order that an appropriate intervention can be arranged.

2. **When there is a danger to somebody else:** A person with a mental illness may engage in behaviour that places others at risk. A patient making credible threats of violence against someone is one such example. The person under threat will be made aware of the threat, as will the Gardaí, who can then investigate it and take the necessary action to protect the threatened person. This is called a Tarasoff Warning, after Titania Tarasoff, who was killed by a man she met at a college dance class. He told his then therapist of his plan and ultimately carried it out by stabbing her. The therapist and his supervisor had written to the college authorities telling them of their concerns for Tarasoff, and the police visited the man who denied that he had stalked Tarasoff. After Tarasoff's death her parents sued the college and the case reached the California Supreme Court, which handed down its decision in 1976. This created the legal duty of a psychiatrist or psychotherapist to warn an identifiable person of a patient's serious threat to harm them. In other words, this principle established that reporting the threat to the police or authorities is not enough, and the potential victim also has to be warned. This is not enshrined in Irish law but it is recognised as an appropriate practice in certain circumstances.

3. **When required by a court:** This most commonly applies to the release of the person's medical records to an independent doctor who will be conducting an examination of an injured party after an accident. Consider a person who says that following a road traffic accident they are consequently suffering from generalised anxiety, and so are taking legal action against the driver of the vehicle. A psychiatrist will be asked to examine the person for an evaluation. They may request the medical records at the time of the accident,

or request that the GP records be provided to them. If this is refused, the court will be asked to make an order for discovery, and if this is granted, as it invariably is, the records must be provided. Any mention of people other than the person taking the case will be redacted, so interviews with family members attending their psychiatrist to provide additional information will be blacked out.

4. **When required by statute:** In Ireland there is a National Cancer Register and a National Self-harm Register, both established by law. This requires the registration of every person with cancer or of each person presenting to emergency departments following an incident of self-harm. The self-harm registrations can range from scratching to high-intent suicide attempts or near-miss suicides. However, the information published in this register is anonymised, and is used only for research to enable better planning of services and to have a greater understanding of what the risk factors are for these conditions. It is not possible to opt out of these registers. They will have been approved by each hospital's ethics committee.

Physical, sexual or emotional abuse

Those with psychiatric illnesses often report historic sexual abuse. In Ireland it is mandatory to report this, even against the wishes of the victim. The position in Ireland differs from that in England and Wales, where there is a degree of discretion in this regard. The rationale behind the mandatory reporting of abuse is that the abuser may still be at large and posing a risk to others. For instance, somebody may claim that their schoolteacher abused them some years ago, and it may be that the teacher is still alive and poses a risk to other young people. Mandatory reporting of abuse is a contentious issue, since some psychiatrists believe that when the abuse occurred in the distant past and the person is no longer any risk to others, e.g. because they are bed-bound in a nursing home, that there should be a degree of discretion. The concerns are that having to report the incident against the patient's wishes may disrupt the doctor-patient relationship and result in the victim feeling disempowered yet again, just as they did when abused. On the other hand, there is concern at the idea of a doctor making an arbitrary decision about whom to report, and that this decision is so grave that it should be left to the Gardaí and child protection agencies This is, to be sure, a hard legislative line to tread. A further legal conundrum is what should happen when a person with an attraction to children attends a psychiatrist for help with their thoughts and feelings. Thoughts are not crimes ordinarily.

A person who is vulnerable because of mental illness and who is currently the victim of physical abuse or neglect may not have the emotional strength to report this to the relevant authorities. It is important to encourage such reporting and to assist the person in so doing. If they are dependent on the abuser for their care and day-to-day activities, the doctor should seek legal advice, and a decision to report the abuse should be made on the basis of the person's capacity to do so. If you know of such a situation you should inform the person's GP or go to the Gardaí.

WHAT IF THE PERSON HAS DIED?

Confidentiality continues after death, and the release of information about a deceased person should occur for only the most serious of reasons. The right of the deceased to have their psychiatric history remain confidential must be balanced by the family's right to information about the deceased, if the person's records are sought. Unless there is a specific legal reason the records are unlikely to be released. Records are most often sought posthumously when there is a contest about a will and it is thought that the deceased did not have the capacity to make a will at the time. They may also be sought in relation to claims of medical negligence and during criminal investigations. In these instances it is common for a judge to rule that these records should be given to the family.

In the course of the person's life, third parties such as spouses or other family members and friends may have been interviewed. In the absence of their permission, the sections of the medical records containing these interviews will be redacted.

Information-sharing with the next of kin

If you are the patient, it is considered best psychiatric practice to share information with those close to you or others agreed by you. The blueprint for best practice in *A Vision for Change* (2006), indicates that, where possible, family members must be kept in the picture and that this must be done 'with care and sensitivity'. Aside from the five unique situations outlined above, if you are a patient, you can refuse to allow information about you to be passed to your next of kin. It is also considered best practice to obtain information about the symptoms you have, your past psychiatric history and background from the next of kin, as well as from you (Casey, 2015). This is because you may have forgotten about previous episodes of illness or the treatments you have had, particularly if you are very ill.

Most people who are being treated for a psychiatric disorder are agreeable to this sharing. When this is refused, it is important to establish why this is. It may be that the family were abusive and, in these circumstances, it would be inappropriate to discuss your information. More commonly the refusal stems from a misunderstanding about what will be provided. You may fear that very specific information about symptoms, or personal matters such as infidelity or prior substance misuse will be passed on to relatives. This is not the case. Usually next of kin have a very specific suite of questions about which they want information. These include:

- the diagnosis
- the cause of your condition, if known
- the treatment
- the prognosis
- the follow-up arrangements if you have been in hospital
- the early signs and symptoms of relapse
- how the family can be of help
- what the family can do in a crisis

If you refuse permission to provide information to your next of kin/carers, you should be reassured by deciding in advance, with your psychiatrist, what can and cannot be discussed (Slade et al., 2007), bearing in mind the above list.

The importance of sharing information to assist in your continuing evaluation and care cannot be emphasised enough. It may help you if you can be present when the information is discussed with the next of kin or with the family. Even after attempts at securing informed consent, you may still refuse to allow specific discussion of your case. This has to be respected unless there are compelling reasons, as discussed above, to act against your wishes. It goes without saying that the relative/next of kin must be told why further information cannot be passed on.

If you are an inpatient, it is most important that your next of kin is told about your impending discharge, and, with your agreement, about such matters as the treatment you are being discharged on and follow-up arrangements with your psychiatrist and other mental health professionals, such as clinical psychologists.

A common complaint by family members is that psychiatrists fob them off and hide behind the cloak of patient confidentiality to avoid disclosing important information to them (Wilson et al., 2015). Even when the patient has given permission it is reported that psychiatrists still refuse to discuss their relative's diagnosis etc. Secrecy, as perceived by family members, is very distressing and amounts to suboptimal practice. There is no reason to withhold information from relatives if the patient consents, unless of course the doctor is of the opinion that the patient is being coerced into agreeing or is from an abusive family.

Over and above the specifics of the person's history of mental health problems, there is nothing in the ethics of confidentiality that prevents a doctor listening to and taking note of someone's concerns about the patient. Indeed, the doctor is arguably legally liable, if a refusal to listen to such concerns results in an adverse outcome for the patient.

Case Vignette

Ms A had been a patient in various psychiatric services around the country. She would stay in one part of the country for a few months and then move to another, to 'make a new start'. In the course of each move she discontinued her medication and would relapse, resulting in frequent compulsory admissions to hospital. She had been diagnosed with schizophrenia 10 years earlier. She was single and her older sister was her only living relative. In her current service she was adhering to treatment and she had stayed for two years, the longest time with any psychiatrist, Dr B. She reluctantly took medication but frequently asked to have vitamins and dietary measures to control her illness. She accepted that medication helped some people but said she wished to try alternative measures as she had read about the dangers of medication. Consequently the psychiatrist got to know her sister who was also her next of kin. She was very pleased her sister was taking medication and on it for so long. Ms A was very well and had a regular job when she advised the psychiatrist that she was planning on moving to another part of the country and she asked for a letter about her illness so that she could give it to the psychiatrist she would find in her new location. The psychiatrist did this and sought her permission to discuss the move with her sister, as Dr B felt this move was ill advised. Ms A absolutely forbade this. She said she was well and had a right to confidentiality. What can the doctor do?

Comment:

This is a complex situation. The patient is clearly well, yet her move, typical of what had happened in the past, is likely to result in her stopping her medication and becoming ill, notwithstanding her stated intention of finding a new psychiatrist in her new location. She has little insight into her illness and into the necessity for medication. She has investigated this and read about alternative approaches to treatment. Her conversation with the psychiatrist suggests that she has capacity – she is currently well and clearly has investigated various treatments other than medication. Her mistrust of this is not apparently driven by delusions but by beliefs about medication that are contained in certain writings.

Ms A currently has capacity since the test is not making the correct decision but understanding the risks/benefits and being able to weigh them. She is correct in that she has a right to confidentiality, and in view of her current capacity Dr B cannot break confidentiality and inform her sister that Ms A intends to move. If Dr B did decide to inform Ms A's sister, she could be reported to the Irish Medical Council, the body that regulates the ethics of medical practice in Ireland, and received a sanction from that body if found guilty.

Note: This is not a real case but is typical of a clinical scenario that touches on issues of capacity and confidentiality.

BIBLIOGRAPHY

The Assisted Decision-Making (Capacity) Act 2015.

Casey, Patricia. 'Beneficence and non-maleficence: confidentiality and carers in psychiatry'. *Irish Journal of Psychological Medicine*. 33, 4. 220306. 2016.

The Mental Health Act 2001.

Mullen, P. 'Facing up to unpalatable evidence for the sake of our patients'. *PLoS Medicine*. 6, 8. E1000112. 2009.

Owens, G. S., Richardson, Genevra, David, A. S. et al. 'Mental capacity to make decisions on treatment in people admitted to psychiatric hospitals: cross-sectional study'. *BMJ*. 337, 7660. 40-42. 2008.

Report of the Expert Group on Mental Health Policy. *A Vision for Change*. Health Service Executive. 2006.

Slade, M., Pinfold, V., Rapaport, J., Bellringer, S., Banerjee, S., Kuipers, E. and Huxley, P. 'Best practice when service users do not consent to sharing information with carers – National multimethod study'. *British Journal of Psychiatry*, 190, 2. pp. 148–55. 2007.

Wilson, L., Pillay, D., Kelly, B. D. and Casey, P. 'Mental health professionals and information sharing: carer perspectives'. *Irish Journal of Medical Science*. 184(4) (2015). 781–90.

USEFUL RESOURCES

HSE. Assisted Decision-Making (Capacity) Act 2015. Explainer video.

Criminal Law Insanity Act 2006.

Department of Health and Children (Ireland) Mental Health Act. Dublin: The Stationery Office. 2001.

RIX Research and Media. 'Mental Capacity Act. Using The Key Principles In Care Planning'. YouTube 18 June 2015.

If only there was more compassion in society

My motivation in writing this piece is broadly to help mental health sufferers and, more specifically, the general public, gain the correct insight into how a person suffering from chronic lifelong mental illness is so unfairly treated to this day in society, and to demonstrate that in order for a more transparent lifestyle to be had by all, what is needed is for the perception of mental illness to change radically, to a much more positive, valued outlook of humanity.

My own experience is that stigma is still a big issue for people who suffer from mental health issues. You are discriminated against in the workplace, sidelined as not competent enough to take on tasks, hence your development within the job is very much restricted, sadly. Similarly, you tend not to be given a chance for promotion opportunities.

The question arises, is the potential employer going to take a chance on someone who suffers from mental ill health? Some employers might but many will not take that chance. Ultimately, I believe, the employers are losing out. The person with sporadically occurring mental health issues can bring so much value to a company, once given a chance. Once their strengths are acknowledged, such as increased empathy, understanding, a strong work ethic, loyalty to the job, less of a tendency to move to other jobs, perhaps, once the person is happy with the status quo in that job and treated fairly and, yes, with compassion from time to time.

With the current pandemic, my experience is that having to restrict my movements does not necessarily increase my levels of hardship. Please allow me to explain. Having been in psychiatric hospitals on numerous occasions and 'locked up' for my own safety, basically, and confined at times, restricted movement does not seem to me like such a big deal. I am kind of used to this pandemic-type lockdown, if you like, in other words being in hospital for prolonged periods.

Everybody can turn this Covid-19 pandemic to their advantage: More quality time to spend with your children/family. More time to read/listen to music and relax, perhaps. More time to be in the now, slow down and watch the beautiful world around us such as the birds and trees, and also time to reflect, which is so critically important to all of us. More time for God – we all need God/spirituality in our lives – prayer can help us through all the difficulties in life that every person will experience. Time to be polite and say 'hello' to others. I often think going down the street, that if you say 'hello' or 'good morning' to someone, you might be the person to lift their spirits that day, perhaps even the only person that day to acknowledge that person, which really means so much!

Honestly, I regard taking lifelong medications as taking my medicine, not a big deal, which ultimately keeps me well and the chemicals in balance. There is no joy in being unwell, I assure you! I know only too well from experience. Hence, I urge fellow mental health sufferers to take your medicine regularly, on time, and never to see it as a big taboo. Remember, most of the population has to take some medicine.

I believe we are all human beings, God's children, and nobody should think less of a mental health sufferer. Rather, in order to help society, the public should pick up a book and read about and inform themselves about mental health issues, in order to help themselves and others. Most importantly, people like me honestly do recover from poor mental health and can have a good life, albeit by maintaining good communication channels (talking therapies) and by taking our meds! Everybody should be mindful of the fact that there are ups and downs for all in life – mental health sufferers are no different from the wider public. Remember also – nobody is beyond suffering from poor mental health in life at some stage. To finish, I really believe, if there is more compassion in society, the world will be a far better place for all!

I rest my case.

INDEX